Second Edition

Documentation Basics
A Guide for the Physical Therapist Assistant

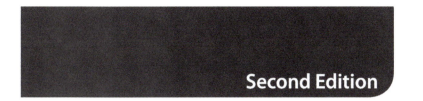

Second Edition

Documentation Basics

A Guide for the
Physical Therapist Assistant

MIA L. ERICKSON, PT, EdD, CHT, ATC
West Virginia University
Department of Human Performance and Applied Exercise Science
Division of Physical Therapy
Morgantown, West Virginia

REBECCA McKNIGHT, PT, MS
Educational Consultant
Powersite, Missouri

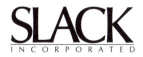

SLACK
INCORPORATED

www.slackbooks.com

ISBN: 978-1-61711-008-5

Copyright © 2012 by SLACK Incorporated

Instructors: *Documentation Basics: A Guide for the Physical Therapist Assistant, Second Edition Instructor's Manual* is also available from SLACK Incorporated. Don't miss this important companion to *Documentation Basics: A Guide for the Physical Therapist Assistant, Second Edition*. To obtain the Instructor's Manual, please visit http://www.efacultylounge.com

The procedures and practices described in this publication should be implemented in a manner consistent with the professional standards set for the circumstances that apply in each specific situation. Every effort has been made to confirm the accuracy of the information presented and to correctly relate generally accepted practices. The authors, editors, and publisher cannot accept responsibility for errors or exclusions or for the outcome of the material presented herein. There is no expressed or implied warranty of this book or information imparted by it. Care has been taken to ensure that drug selection and dosages are in accordance with currently accepted/recommended practice. Off-label uses of drugs may be discussed. Due to continuing research, changes in government policy and regulations, and various effects of drug reactions and interactions, it is recommended that the reader carefully review all materials and literature provided for each drug, especially those that are new or not frequently used. Some drugs or devices in this publication have clearance for use in a restricted research setting by the Food and Drug and Administration or FDA. Each professional should determine the FDA status of any drug or device prior to use in their practice.

Any review or mention of specific companies or products is not intended as an endorsement by the author or publisher.

SLACK Incorporated uses a review process to evaluate submitted material. Prior to publication, educators or clinicians provide important feedback on the content that we publish. We welcome feedback on this work.

Published by: SLACK Incorporated
                  6900 Grove Road
                  Thorofare, NJ 08086 USA
                  Telephone: 856-848-1000
                  Fax: 856-848-6091
                  www.slackbooks.com

Contact SLACK Incorporated for more information about other books in this field or about the availability of our books from distributors outside the United States.

Library of Congress Cataloging-in-Publication Data

Erickson, Mia L.
  Documentation basics : a guide for the physical therapist assistant / Mia L. Erickson, Rebecca McKnight. -- 2nd ed.
      p. ; cm.
  Includes bibliographical references and index.
  ISBN 978-1-61711-008-5 (alk. paper)
  I. McKnight, Rebecca, II. Title.
  [DNLM: 1. Medical Records. 2. Physical Therapy Specialty--organization & administration. 3. Allied Health Personnel. WB 460]
  LC classification not assigned
  615.8'2--dc23
                        2012007230

For permission to reprint material in another publication, contact SLACK Incorporated. Authorization to photocopy items for internal, personal, or academic use is granted by SLACK Incorporated provided that the appropriate fee is paid directly to Copyright Clearance Center. Prior to photocopying items, please contact the Copyright Clearance Center at 222 Rosewood Drive, Danvers, MA 01923 USA; phone: 978-750-8400; web site: www.copyright.com; email: info@copyright.com

Printed in the United States of America.

Last digit is print number: 10   9   8   7   6   5   4   3   2

CONTENTS

Instructors: *Documentation Basics: A Guide for the Physical Therapist Assistant, Second Edition Instructor's Manual* is also available from SLACK Incorporated. Don't miss this important companion to *Documentation Basics: A Guide for the Physical Therapist Assistant, Second Edition*. To obtain the Instructor's Manual, please visit http://www.efacultylounge.com

ACKNOWLEDGMENTS

I would like to acknowledge the PTA program at Allegany College of Maryland and the Class of 2002 for helping me to realize the need for this book. In addition, I would like to express my sincerest thanks to the editing team at SLACK Incorporated for working with us. To my wonderful family, you are the light of my life, and I am so thankful to have your love and support in all of my adventures. Lastly, I cannot say thank you enough to Becky for being a great coauthor.

Mia Erickson

I would like to acknowledge the many PTA graduates from Ozarks Technical Community College who were my "guinea pigs" and helped me gain a clearer picture of how to communicate documentation issues to students. I would also like to thank Mia for her patience and willingness to allow me to continue to develop the work we started. Most importantly, I would like to thank my husband and my daughter Jessica (the last of six and the only one still at home) for putting up with me as I "obsessed" over this project. Finally, I must continue to thank my God and King, Jesus Christ, for his continual blessings, one of which is the honor of coauthoring this text.

Becky McKnight

ABOUT THE AUTHORS

Mia L. Erickson, PT, EdD, CHT, ATC is currently an Associate Professor and Co-Academic Coordinator of Clinical Education at West Virginia University. She has a bachelor's degree in secondary education and athletic training from West Virginia University. She received a master of science degree in physical therapy from the University of Indianapolis in 1996 and completed her doctoral degree in education at West Virginia University in 2002. She participates in clinical practice in Fairmont, West Virginia in outpatient hand and upper extremity rehabilitation.

Rebecca McKnight, PT, MS received her bachelor's of science degree in physical therapy from St. Louis University in 1992 and her post-professional master of science degree from Rocky Mountain University of Health Professions in 1999. Rebecca taught at Ozarks Technical Community College for 14 years, serving as program director for 9 of those years. Ms. McKnight is an active member of the American Physical Therapy Association (APTA), and is a former chair of the PTA Educators Special Interest Group of the Education Section. She has spoken at many national meetings on Physical Therapist Assistant curriculum design and programmatic assessment. She is the 2009 recipient of the F.A. Davis Award for Outstanding Physical Therapist Assistant Educator.

Rebecca has recently begun a consulting business with her husband (Reach Consulting) and provides consultation related to curriculum design, development, and assessment to physical therapist assistant programs nationwide.

PREFACE

With a new, more contemporary look, the second edition of *Documentation Basics: A Guide for the Physical Therapist Assistant* is similar in layout to the first edition. The introductory information is provided first, followed by student practice sections. The book also includes some introductory information on reimbursement in different settings, legal and ethical issues associated with documentation, and a chapter dedicated to helping you provide documentation examples for students in many areas of physical therapy practice.

In the second edition, we have shifted the language from the Nagi disablement terminology to terminology from the *International Classification of Functioning, Disability, and Health*, or the ICF. Instead of using a term like *functional limitation*, we have included *activity limitation* and *participation restriction*. We increased the emphasis on linking impairments to function and the need to be descriptive in how the interventions have influenced both impairments and function. There are many updated examples of how we can show "skill" in our interventions. We also expanded the section on electronic documentation. While we have kept the SOAP structure for documentation, there is discussion on how this format lends itself to the electronic record and the use of templates. We also divided the "practice" section into four stand-alone chapters so that students would be able to see the unique characteristics of each of the four parts of a SOAP note.

In addition, we have some exciting new information. There is an example of a more contemporary use of the problem-oriented medical record. There is a small discussion on documentation in early intervention and school-based physical therapy, as well as new pediatric examples throughout. We also expanded the chapters on reimbursement to include Medicare Parts C and D, along with cash-based and pro bono services. There is also an addition that discusses the importance of the PT initial documentation under prospective payment systems and how it informs the case-mix assignment. The chapter on legal issues now includes HIPAA Privacy and Security Rules. We also provided a few new SNAC examples, additional forms and templates, and a sample PT evaluation completed on a template for a patient who obtained physical therapy through direct access. We have also updated the references and provided ways that students can locate up-to-date information in such a rapidly changing area.

Chapter 4 is new and this is my favorite. It is a discussion on how the PTA uses the initial PT documentation. It blends the initial documentation with PTA clinical decision-making as it outlines a process for the PTA to identify pertinent information and use it to prepare for and work with the patient. It provides information to guide the PTA in what equipment to gather, what measures to perform, what interventions to perform, and then how to put it all together in the documentation.

Finally, we have provided instructor resources including teaching tips, answers to review questions and application exercises, sample notes for the SNAC section, exam questions, and slides. We hope you like the new version and materials as much as we do.

Mia L. Erickson, PT, EdD, CHT, ATC

Chapter 1
Physical Therapy and Disablement

Mia L. Erickson, PT, EdD, CHT, ATC

CHAPTER OBJECTIVES

After reading this chapter, the student will be able to do the following:

1. Describe how the definitions of health and disability have changed throughout history.
2. Define disablement.
3. Define terminology used in the *International Classification of Functioning, Disability, and Health* (ICF) and terminology used in the Nagi framework.
4. Differentiate between impairment, functional limitation, and disability.
5. Compare and contrast the ICF and the Nagi framework.
6. Differentiate between impairment, activity limitation, and participation restriction.
7. Differentiate between activities of daily living (ADL) and instrumental activities of daily living (IADL).
8. Define documentation.
9. Describe the relationship between documentation and disablement.

DEFINING HEALTH AND DISABILITY

A traditional approach to defining a person's health comes from the biomedical model in which *health* means free or absent from disease.[1] In this biomedical model, there is heavy emphasis on treating and curing a person's disease and little emphasis on how the disease affects the person's ability to function within society on a day-to-day basis.[1] In the 1950s and 1960s, government agencies began programs to dispense funds to individuals with disabilities caused by disease or injury; for example, Social Security, Veteran Compensation, and Workers' Compensation. However, differing definitions of disability created controversy as agencies determined the amount of money an individual was to be awarded.[2]

More contemporary models have defined health in terms that go beyond the patient's medical diagnosis or disease. Across the country and throughout the world, individuals and groups have developed models that acknowledge the importance of societal, psychological, and physical functioning in the presence of disease.[1] Rather than placing the measure of health on the disease process itself, more recent models have shifted toward examining an individual's ability to carry out necessary life tasks and function within society. The consequences of disease as they pertain to the relationship between body structures, ability to carry out tasks, and ability to function within society have become known as *disablement*.[3]

Traditionally, physical therapists have been interested in measuring patient impairments or deviations from normal anatomical, physiological, mental, or psychological structure or function.[4] However, a more contemporary approach in physical therapy practice is to incorporate disablement or examine how the patient functions within his or her environment. Physical therapists assess function through observation of patient performance of functional tasks or through patient self-report questionnaires. Documenting patient function at the initial examination and then again through periodic reassessments is important for third-party payment or reimbursement. Impairment measures such as strength, range of motion, and balance are still widely used, but it is important that these impairment measures are linked to disablement or patient function. The purpose of this chapter is to introduce you to common disablement frameworks.

Erickson M, McKnight R. *Documentation Basics:*
A Guide for the Physical Therapist Assistant, Second Edition (pp. 1-8)
© 2012 SLACK Incorporated

Figure 1-1. Overview of the Nagi disablement framework.

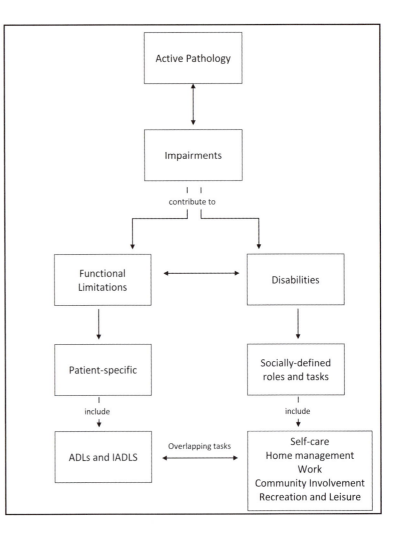

After reading, you will have a sense of what aspects of disablement should be included as well as their importance. Throughout this text, you will be introduced to incorporating disablement into your clinical documentation.

There are several major disablement models, or conceptual frameworks, used to describe health and disability. The two that will be described here are (1) the Nagi framework,[2] developed by Saad Nagi, and (2) the ICF,[5] developed by the World Health Organization (WHO).

THE NAGI FRAMEWORK

The Nagi framework was developed in the 1960s by sociologist Saad Nagi.[2] Nagi constructed a conceptual framework using the terms active pathology, impairment, functional limitation, and disability (Figure 1-1). Nagi's model and terminology were used in the *Guide to Physical Therapist Practice* to provide a framework for practicing therapists.[4] Nagi's model provided the following terminology and definitions.[2]

Pathology is the interruption or interference with normal process and the simultaneous body efforts to heal itself or regain a normal state. This is often referred to as the disease itself. The pathology occurs at the cellular, tissue, or organ level and is often the patient's medical diagnosis.[4] Medical management and physician interventions are often directed at reducing the active pathology. Examples of active pathologies include osteoporosis, Parkinson disease, and radius fracture.

Impairments are losses or abnormalities of an anatomical, physiological, mental, or emotional nature. Impairments are deviations from normal. They generally result from the pathology and comprise signs and symptoms of a specific pathology.[2] In physical therapy, common impairments include limited range of motion, muscle weakness, impaired balance, decreased sensation, and limited circulation.

Functional limitations are abnormalities or limitations in an individual's ability to carry out a meaningful action, task, or activity.[2,4] The *Guide to Physical Therapist Practice* describes 2 types of functional abilities. First, there are those associated with basic ADLs, such as moving in bed, transferring from one surface to another, rising from a chair, ambulating, dressing, bathing, etc. In addition, there are activities associated with more complex independent living and community-dwelling skills. These more complex behaviors are known as IADLs and include community ambulation activities, such as going to a grocery store, bank, or restaurant.[4] Impairments often lead to functional limitations. For instance, an individual with limited shoulder range of motion (impairment) might be unable to reach into an overhead cabinet or have difficulty donning a shirt (functional limitations). A patient with decreased quadriceps strength (impairment) might have difficulty ambulating without assistance (functional limitation). Functional limitations are patient-specific. In other words, limitations will vary depending on the individual's lifestyle and functional demands. Read the following scenarios:

> There are two patients, both 65-year-old females who have knee osteoarthritis. Patient 1 lives in a single-level house and enjoys gardening. Her primary complaint is difficulty kneeling. Patient 2 lives in a multilevel townhouse with 2 flights of stairs. Her chief complaint is difficulty ascending and descending stairs.

> In patient 1, the functional limitation is kneeling and for patient 2, the functional limitation is stair climbing. Both patients have the same pathology and likely have similar impairments, but their functional limitations are tasks that are specific to the individual. These are based on functional demands of their lifestyles and life activities.

Functional limitations relate to the fourth aspect of the Nagi framework—disability. The most direct way that impairments contribute to disabilities is through functional limitations.[2] According to the Nagi framework, *disability* is the inability or limitation in performing socially defined roles and tasks that would normally be expected of an individual within a given culture or environment.[2] Unlike functional limitations, which are patient-specific, disabilities are roles or tasks that have been socially defined as "normal" for a given population. These roles and tasks are organized by life activities including (1) self-care, (2) home management, (3) work, (4) community involvement, and (5) recreation or leisure.[4]

Because disability in Nagi's model is socially constructed rather than centered on impairments or functional limitations alone, dissimilar pathologies, impairments, and functional limitations can produce similar disabilities. Furthermore, individuals with similar impairments and functional limitations might have differing degrees of disability depending on their functional demands. Let's look at two more examples:

> Patient 1: A 32-year-old male computer programmer with shoulder impingement syndrome has pain when reaching overhead. The patient is able to perform normal work duties because he spends most of the day at his computer.

> Patient 2: A 45-year-old male mechanic with shoulder impingement also has pain when reaching overhead. This patient is unable to work due to his inability to reach overhead because he spends most of his day with his arms in an elevated position.

In these examples, both patients have the same pathology and functional limitation—reaching. But they have different levels of disability due to their work demands.

Nagi[2] provided 3 factors that influence an individual's perception of his or her degree of disability. These include (1) the individual's situation and his or her reaction to the situation; (2) the reactions of others, such as family, friends, associates, and coworkers; and (3) environmental barriers.

There is often overlap between an individual's functional limitations and his or her disabilities, and this can be a point of confusion. An individual could be limited in a task that has also been determined appropriate for his or her age or environment. Let's look at an example:

> A 24-year-old male is involved in a motor vehicle accident and sustains an L2–L3 incomplete spinal cord injury. Some of his lower extremity muscles are still intact, and the patient learns to ambulate independently with ankle–foot orthoses and Lofstrand crutches.

In this example, the individual is limited functionally due to the lower extremity weakness. He must wear assistive devices, and he probably has an abnormal gait pattern that requires high energy expenditure. One would also say that ambulation is an appropriate, socially defined task for a 24-year-old male. Therefore, in this example, limited ambulation is both a functional limitation and a disability. Now, if the same individual can only walk short distances with the assistive devices due to poor endurance and he uses a wheelchair for longer distances, the degree of disability increases.

THE ICF

The ICF, originally known as the *International Classification of Impairments, Disabilities, and Handicaps* (ICIDH), was endorsed by the Fifty-fourth World Health Assembly and released in 2001. The ICF provides a uniform, standard language for describing an individual's health and health-related state that moves beyond his or her diagnosis.[5] The ICF also accounts for facilitators and barriers to function that might appear in a patient's surroundings.[6] These things include ramps and handrails. The individual's health or health-related state is described in terms of function and disability. What the individual *can* do is known as functioning, or the positive aspects of health. What the individual *cannot* do is known as disability, or the negative aspects of health (Figure 1-2).[5]

Function and disability compose Part 1 of the ICF. Part 1 is further divided into 2 components, (1) Body Functions (physiological function) and Body Structures (anatomical structures) and (2) Activities (individual-specific tasks) and Participation (life roles; see Figure 1-2). In categorizing an individual's health according to the ICF, a health care provider would describe body structures and functions that are intact (known as *positive aspects*) as well as those that are not intact (known as *negative aspects*). Any deviation(s) from normal body structure and/or function are known as impairments. For the activities and participa-

Figure 1-2. Overview of the *International Classification of Functioning, Disability, and Health*.[1] The string of boxes on the left represent the positive aspects of the health state, or condition. The string of boxes on the right represent deviations from normal, or negative aspects of health.

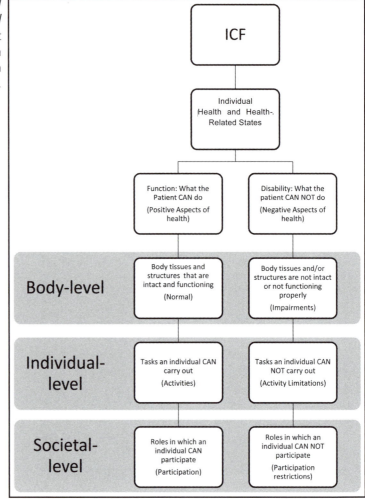

tion component, the examiner identifies functional tasks that the individual can do (known as *activities*) and those he or she cannot do (known as *activity limitations*). The examiner also identifies life roles that the individual can carry out (*participation*) and cannot carry out (known as *participation restrictions*; see Figure 1-2).[5] The activities and participation component of the ICF is one of the biggest differences between the Nagi framework and the ICF.

Because activities and participation are often dependent on the setting, or context, in which the patient functions, the creators of the ICF have included Part 2, Contextual Factors. Part 2 includes environmental and personal factors that affect the individual's functioning and disability. Environmental factors are external factors, either immediate or global, that affect the individual's ability to participate in society. These might be *facilitators*, which enhance participation, or *barriers*, which deter participation. Environmental factors include things like physical structures, such as ramps, stairs, or curbs. Personal factors are those that are unique to the individual, such as attitude, mood, or family support (Figure 1-3).[5] Integration of the contextual factors

is another important difference between the Nagi framework and the ICF.

The ICF is part of a family of classifications created by the WHO, known as the WHO Family of International Classifications (FIC). The WHO-FIC also includes the *International Classification of Diseases* (ICD). The ICD is a classification system for medical diagnoses and diseases.[5] At the time of this publication, the United States health care system was using the ICD-9, or 9th revision. At some time in the future, there will be a shift to the ICD-10, or 10th revision. The 2 classification systems are meant to complement each other in that the ICD provides a catalog of medical diagnoses, diseases, disorders, and health conditions and the ICF provides corresponding information on function and disability. Used together, they provide a broader picture of the individual's health.[7] In 2008, the American Physical Therapy Association's (APTA) House of Delegates voted to endorse the ICF and, as a result, future APTA publications, documents, and communications will incorporate ICF language (Example 1-1).[8] As the profession transitions from the Nagi framework to the ICF, there will likely be some issues with terminology among students

	Part 1: Functioning and Disability		Part 2: Contextual Factors	
Components	Body Functions and Structures	Activities and Participation	Environmental Factors	Personal Factors
Domains	Body functions Body structures	Life areas (tasks, actions)	External influences on functioning and disability	Internal influences on functioning and disability
Constructs	Change in body functions (physiological) Change in body structures (anatomical)	Capacity -- Executing tasks in a standard environment Performance -- Executing tasks in the current environment	Facilitating or hindering impact of features (attributes) of the physical, social, and attitudinal world	Impact of attributes of the person
Positive aspect	Functional and structural integrity Functioning	Activities Participation	Facilitators	not applicable
Negative aspect	Impairment Disability	Activity limitation Participation restriction	Barriers/hindrances	not applicable

Figure 1-3. The *International Classification of Functioning, Disability, and Health* (ICF)[5] from the World Health Organization. (Reprinted with permission from the World Health Organization.)

Example 1-1

The following definitions have been endorsed by the WHO as part of the ICF:[5]
- *Functioning* is an umbrella term that includes all body functions, activities, and participation.
- *Disability* serves as an umbrella term for impairments, activity limitations, and participation restrictions.
- *Body functions* are physiological functions of the body (including psychological function).
- *Body structures* are anatomical bodily structures, such as organs, limbs, etc.
- *Impairments* are problems with body functions (physiological, psychological) or structures, such as a deviation or loss.
- *Activity* is the execution of a task or activity by an individual.
- *Activity limitations* are difficulties that might be encountered by an individual who is attempting to complete a task or carry out an activity.
- *Participation* is involvement in a life situation, such as work or school.
- *Participation restrictions* are problems an individual might face while involved in life situations.
- *Contextual factors* are the complete factors that make up a person's life and living, including his or her background.
- *Environmental factors* are the physical, social, and attitudinal environments in which people live and carry out their lives. These include things immediate to the individual, such as his or her home or workplace and the larger social context, such as government agencies designed to assist people with disabilities.
- *Personal factors* are factors specific to the individual and his or her background. These include things like age, gender, social habits, health habits, upbringing, coping strategies, etc.

or recent graduates and clinicians who have not practiced using the ICF. The overview of the models in this text can help with understanding the differences in the language.

PHYSICAL THERAPY AND DISABLEMENT: GOING BEYOND IMPAIRMENT

Both the Nagi model and the ICF provide frameworks for examining the relationship between disease or injury, impairments, function, and participation within society. They provide a mechanism for exploring the impact of disease or injury on an individual's day-to-day life. Consideration of disablement when working with patients helps therapists to realize more complex functional and social issues that patients face.

Individuals in need of physical therapy services often have a disease or injury with resulting impairments and functional loss that are illuminated by the physical therapy examination. Impairments are often limitations in range of motion, strength, and balance. But to see how the patient's ability to function has been compromised, the examination must go beyond the impairment level. It is our responsibility to understand how impairments affect the patient's day-to-day activities and participation in a variety of settings and situations. Therefore, the physical therapist's examination of patient function should include things like hygiene and self-care; home management (yard work, household cleaning); ability to work, go to school, or play; ability to participate in community activities (going to the grocery store or bank); and ability to participate in recreational activities. By understanding an individual's impairments as well as his or her activity limitations and participation restrictions, we can better understand the degree of disability associated with the pathology for each patient.

DISABLEMENT AND DOCUMENTATION

Documentation, otherwise known as medical record keeping, has been defined as "any entry into the patient/client record, such as a(n) consultation report, initial examination report, progress note, flow sheet/checklist, that identifies the care/service provided, re-examination, or summation of care."[4(p686)] Redgate and Foto[9] indicated that complete documentation also includes the physician prescription(s) and certification(s), communication with other care providers, copies of exercise programs or patient instructions, and any other disciplines' notes or comments that support the interventions.

As you will read in subsequent chapters, documentation will serve many purposes, such as maintaining data collected on patients and providing information to other health care providers, to name a few. There are also many styles and formats for physical therapy records. Regardless of the purpose of your documentation or the style that you are using, your documentation should reflect disablement. One reason for integrating disablement concepts in physical therapy is to achieve consistency in terminology for practice, reimbursement, and research. This begins by way of consistency in our terminology used in documentation, because our notes are the sole record of the episode of care provided to each patient or client. Another reason is to show the reader how the patient's pathology and impairments influence his or her daily life.

Disablement concepts serve as a foundation for this text. Throughout the chapters, you will be reminded of 3 important disablement concepts that should be integrated into your clinical documentation:

1. Your documentation should reflect not only patient impairments but also activity limitations and participation restrictions.
2. You should be describing *how* the patient's impairments relate or contribute to his or her activity limitations and participation restrictions.
3. Documentation should explain how physical therapy interventions are bringing about changes in impairments and function that relate to the patient's therapy goals.

REFERENCES

1. Mandich A, Miller L, Law M. Outcomes in evidence-based practice. In: Law M, ed. *Evidence-Based Rehabilitation: A Guide to Practice.* Thorofare, NJ: SLACK Incorporated; 2002:50–69.
2. Nagi S. Disability concepts revisited: implications for prevention. In: Pope AM, Tarlov AR, eds. *Disability in America: Toward a National Agenda for Prevention.* Washington, DC: National Academy Press; 1991:309–327.
3. Quinn L, Gordon J. *Functional Outcomes: Documentation for Rehabilitation.* St. Louis, Mo: Saunders; 2003.
4. American Physical Therapy Association. *The Guide to Physical Therapist Practice.* Alexandria, Va: American Physical Therapy Association; 2001. Available at: guidetoptpractice.apta.org. Accessed February 18, 2012.
5. World Health Organization. *The International Classification of Functioning, Disability, and Health.* Geneva, Switzerland: World Health Organization; 2001. Available at: http://whqlibdoc.who.int/publications/2001/9241545429.pdf. Accessed February 24, 2011.
6. World Health Organization. WHO publishes new guidelines to measure health [press release]. Available at: http://www.who.int/inf-pr-2001/en/pr2001-48.html. Accessed November 15, 2001.
7. Bemis-Dougherty A. Practice matters: what is the ICF? *PT Magazine.* 2009;17(1):44, 46.
8. American Physical Therapy Association. APTA endorses World Health Organization ICF model. Available at: http://www.apta.org/AM/Template.cfm?Section=Home&TEMPLATE=/CM/ContentDisplay.cfm&CONTENTID=50081. Accessed February 24, 2011.
9. Redgate N, Foto M. Pay by the rules: avoid Medicare audits and reduce payment denials with a sound strategy and proper documentation. *Physical Therapy Products.* October–November 2003:28–30.

REVIEW QUESTIONS

1. How is a person's health determined today as opposed to 5 decades ago?

2. In your own words, describe disablement.

3. Why is there a need for disablement models today? Why are they important to you?

4. What are the 2 major disablement models today?

5. Complete the table below using terminology from the ICF and the Nagi framework. Use the following terms: *pathology, impairment, functional limitation, disability, activity limitation,* and *participation restriction.*

	ICF	Nagi
A patient's medical diagnosis		
Loss or deviation from normal anatomy and/or physiology		
Difficulties encountered when an individual attempts to carry out a single task		
The ability to participate in a normal life role is compromised by disease or injury		
The result of impairments and functional limitations		
Encompasses impairments, activity limitations, and participation restrictions		

6. What is the difference between ADL and IADL? Give 3 examples of each.

7. How are impairments and functional limitations related?

8. How are impairments, functional limitations, and disabilities related?

9. How should physical therapy documentation integrate disablement concepts?

10. On what disablement model will all future APTA documents be based?

APPLICATION EXERCISES

I. Determine whether the following are pathology (P), impairment (I), functional limitation (FL), or disability (D) according to the Nagi framework.

    _____ Rotator cuff tendinitis

    _____ Decreased sensation

    _____ Impaired balance

    _____ Cerebrovascular accident

    _____ Inability to transfer out of bed

    _____ Inability to drive without hand controls

    _____ Inability to rise from a chair without assistance

    _____ Below-knee amputation

    _____ Limited gait distance

    _____ Inability to work

II. Of the above, which could be functional limitations and disabilities, depending on the patient? Why?

III. Determine whether the following are body structure (BS), body function (BF), impairment (I), activity limitation (AL), or participation restriction (PR) according to the ICF.

    _____ Taking a bath

    _____ Going to school

    _____ Brushing teeth

    _____ Walking in the community

    _____ Going to the grocery store

    _____ Ascending and descending stairs

    _____ Turning a knob

    _____ Writing

    _____ Working

    _____ Bathing

IV. Read the following scenarios and determine the patient's functional limitations and disabilities.

1. You are working with a 70-year-old male who had a total hip replacement 3 weeks ago. He is now able to move in and out of the bed independently, transfer to a chair placed at the bedside, and ambulate 25 feet with a standard walker. He wants to return to driving, golfing, and playing with his grandchildren.

2. You are working with a 10-year-old female in the school system. Her medical diagnosis (pathology) is cerebral palsy, spastic diplegia type. You have been working on ambulating up and down the stairs (which she can perform with minimum assist of 1, a quad cane, and a handrail) and increasing the speed of her gait. At the present time, she leaves her classes early so that she can make it to the next one on time, and she uses the elevator rather than the stairs.

3. Your patient is a 15 year old who sustained a traumatic closed head injury in a motorcycle accident. He is confused and disoriented, and he requires constant supervision for his safety. He can walk and get in and out of bed with supervision. He can also ascend and descend stairs with supervision.

Chapter 2

Reasons for Documenting

Mia L. Erickson, PT, EdD, CHT, ATC

CHAPTER OBJECTIVES

After reading this chapter, the student will be able to do the following:

1. List reasons for documenting.
2. Describe types of patient data found in a medical record.
3. Explain the clinical decision-making process.
4. Explain the physical therapist assistant's (PTA) role in the clinical decision-making process.
5. Describe criteria for medical necessity and skilled care.
6. Differentiate between skilled care and maintenance therapy.
7. Realize the importance of accurate documentation.

Imagine that you are working as a PTA in a small outpatient clinic. For the last 6 weeks, you and your supervising physical therapist (PT) have been working with a 35-year-old male who was recently involved in a motor vehicle accident. He sustained a concussion and multiple fractures including the left femur and radius. Initially, he was unable to bear weight through either extremity and required a wheelchair as his primary mode of mobility. He had significant loss in range of motion (ROM) and was unable to perform self-care, home/community mobility, and work activities. He has been making excellent progress and is now able to walk using one crutch and has resumed most of his normal ADLs. The PT with whom you are working receives a call from the patient's insurance company stating that they are going to deny payment for physical therapy services. In order to have additional therapy services approved, the clinic must submit adequate documentation showing that further skilled services are medically necessary.

LEGAL AND ETHICAL RESPONSIBILITY

As a PTA, documentation will be one of the most important things you do. In health care, documentation has always provided a legal record of care, facilitated communication among health care providers, and served as a source of information for clinical research.[1] Both state and federal laws mandate recording health care provided to an individual. Facilities and organizations providing components of the patient/client management model have policies pertaining to documentation.

Medical records are legal documents, and any entry you make into the medical record becomes part of that legal document. Therefore, it is important that your documentation is accurate, legible, and that it depicts the patient's condition and intervention appropriately and completely. Be aware that a patient's medical records can be subpoenaed and used as evidence in a variety of legal matters. These include motor vehicle accidents, workers' compensation or disability claims, and malpractice suits brought against you or other health care providers. In malpractice lawsuits, documentation is the clinician's first line of defense. Good documentation can stop a lawsuit in its tracks, and poor documentation can be "powerful evidence in support of a suit, even when the accusations are frivolous."[2(p30)] Consider the following as a rule of thumb: "If it isn't documented, it didn't happen."

As the health care delivery system in the United States has evolved over the last decades, third-party payment (ie, reimbursement from insurance companies) has become another reason for providing documentation of patient care. Reimbursement from third-party payers is directly

Erickson M, McKnight R. *Documentation Basics:*
A Guide for the Physical Therapist Assistant, Second Edition (pp. 9-18)
© 2012 SLACK Incorporated

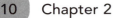

linked with documentation and its ability to show the need for physical therapy services provided. Medical record documentation became a requirement for reimbursement by government agencies such as Medicare and Medicaid as early as 1966.[1] Soon after that, Medicare began a restructuring process and started requiring rehabilitation facilities to not only maintain documentation but also to submit the records for review by Medicare auditors. The purpose of these reviews was to determine whether physical therapy services provided to Medicare beneficiaries met requirements for reimbursement. This decision prompted some of the early literature in our profession in the area of documentation. Consider the patient case on the previous page. Continuation of his physical therapy benefits is based largely on how well the clinicians have documented his improvement and the need for ongoing services.

In addition to legal obligations and reimbursement, maintaining accurate, timely, well-written patient records is considered one of your ethical duties as a PTA. The *Standards of Ethical Conduct for the Physical Therapist Assistant* states, "Physical therapist assistants shall ensure that documentation for their interventions accurately reflects the nature and extent of services provided."[3(p2)] In addition to the legal requirements and ethical responsibilities associated with documentation, PTs and PTAs document to record patient data and care provided. These data, however, must be further elaborated upon so that records show that care is both reasonable and necessary as well as demonstrate clinical decision making.

RECORD PATIENT DATA

One of the primary reasons for documenting physical therapy services is to maintain a record of patient data. These data should reflect the entire episode of patient care, from start to finish, beginning with an initial examination performed by the PT and ending with a discharge summary. During the initial examination, the PT collects and records data pertaining to the patient's current condition. This includes both subjective and objective information. Subjective information is what the patient says pertaining to his or her condition. History of the current condition, mechanism of injury, date of onset, and history of a similar problem are all examples of subjective information gathered during the initial examination. Other subjective information collected at this point should include a thorough medical history, a review of the patient's living situation, chief complaints (including his or her functional limitations and activities that he or she is unable to complete or perform), and his or her goals for physical therapy.

In addition to subjective information, documented data should include results from objective tests and measurements. Examples of these types of objective data include measurements of ROM, strength, sensation, girth, bal-

ance, and functional status (eg, walking, transferring, and performing activities such as self-care and home management). Objective data are obtained through tests and measurements performed by the PT or through patient self-reported pain and disability questionnaires (see Chapter 8). Objective data are used to identify and examine the extent of the patient's impairments, activity limitations, and participation restrictions.

A record of the patient's functional status also provides particularly valuable information regarding the effects of the disease or injury on the patient's normal activities and lifestyle. Furthermore, individuals reviewing medical records deem the patient's functional status as being more meaningful than documentation of impairments alone. Though impairment data are necessary, documenting function, including activity limitations and participation restrictions, provides reviewers with specific contextual information regarding the impact of injury on the patient's lifestyle.

Both subjective and objective data provide PTs and PTAs with baseline measurements to which future measurements can be compared.[4] Information taken from the patient, as well as objective measurements, is not only documented during the initial examination but also during subsequent physical therapy sessions. These data are recorded in the form of treatment notes, interim notes, progress notes, or, in the case of discharge from physical therapy services, in a discharge summary. In any event, any subsequent data collected after the initial examination should be recorded and compared to that found in the initial examination. This allows the medical record to reflect both subjective (patient comments) and objective (data from tests/measurements) changes in the patient's status.

Records of patient data are important to other individuals involved in the patient's care. Health care providers such as physicians, nurses, occupational and speech therapists, case managers, etc are often interested in a patient's status and therefore might examine physical therapy documentation. Physicians might be interested in how far a patient can ambulate prior to deciding on discharge from the hospital. Nurses might be interested in a patient's ability to transfer; case managers might want to examine equipment needs or return-to-work status. Therefore, documentation serves as a useful tool for facilitating communication across disciplines. In addition to other health care providers, third-party payers are interested in records of patient data. Communication with third-party payers through appropriate documentation has been determined to be the "key to securing reimbursement."[5(p14)]

Accurate records of patient data also aid in our ability to analyze and study patient outcomes. Outcomes are defined as the end result of patient/client management.[6] Collection of outcomes data is a growing area in physical therapy that is necessary for evidence-based practice. For example, analysis of patient outcomes can allow us to determine the effectiveness of physical therapy interventions. A goal of the *Guide to Physical Therapist Practice* is to standardize terminology among physical therapy providers.[6] Use of standard terminology when documenting patient data can facilitate outcomes data collection.[7]

RECORD PATIENT CARE

Your documentation will also serve as a record of the care you provided to your patients. Direct and indirect interventions should be recorded. Interventions recorded include those related to direct patient care such as modalities, physical agents (ice, heat), massage, stretching exercises, strengthening exercises, gait training, transfer training, etc. Other interventions include education provided to the patient as well as the patient's understanding and his or her response to the education. Phone calls, relevant conversations regarding the patient, and collaboration with other providers, including the PT, must also be documented as part of the patient's record.

Documented interventions, whether direct or indirect, serve to support treatment that was billed for a given date of service. Third-party payers may perform an audit to assure that the treatment provided and billed is supported by the clinician's documentation. Billing for services not adequately documented is unethical. PTs and PTAs must make every attempt to accurately record and justify services that were billed. Inaccurate or incomplete documentation that does not support daily charges may be construed as fraud or abuse and must be avoided.

Accurately recording patient care is also necessary where computer billing and documentation packages are integrated. In these situations, the patient's charges are generated based on the interventions the therapist provided and documented in the day's note. Incomplete or inaccurate documentation may generate too many or too few charges to the patient's account. Additionally, a patient may be charged for a service not provided. Again, these inconsistencies can prompt an audit, which can result in fines, repayment, or accusations of abuse or fraud, so it is very important that the record accurately reflect all aspects of the care provided to the patient.

Another reason for documenting patient care is to keep a record for other therapists in the event of your absence. In the event of an emergency where you are unable to come to work, another PT or PTA should be able to pick up the record and work with the patient. This maintains consistency of care across providers.

In addition to specific patient care provided, it is important to document the patient's response to treatment. This can be done in a variety of ways. Thinking in terms of disablement, response to treatment should provide information as to how the interventions you provide are positively or negatively influencing the patient's impairments and functional status. For example, a PT could record the following:

> Dynamic balance training and lower extremity strengthening exercise have allowed the patient to improve balance as measured by the Berg Balance Test and patient is now at less risk for falls.

In this example, the PT documented the patient's overall response to treatment in terms of impairments (improved balance) and function (less risk of falls). Consider this example written by a PTA:

> Upon arrival patient was complaining of 6/10 pain in the buttock and leg and was having difficulty sitting. Following modalities and extension exercises, the pain decreased to 3/10 and was no longer radiating down the leg. The patient was able to walk without pain.

In documenting response to treatment in this manner, the note reflects how the interventions influenced both the impairments and function. It can help the PT decide whether the treatment is effective or not. Being specific in the patient's response can show a third-party payer how the patient is improving and how the treatment is influencing impairments and function.

Documenting response to treatment can serve as a record of unexpected events that may have taken place and your response. For example, a patient returns for a therapy visit and has increased soreness after performing his home exercise program. The PTA makes adjustments within the plan of care to lower the exercise intensity. Patient complaints should be documented and the therapist actions in response to the patient's complaints should also be documented. The therapist's response to an adverse event may not always be directed toward the patient. For example, a PT goes to see a patient 4 weeks post total knee arthroplasty for a re-evaluation in the patient's home. The patient is complaining of severe knee pain, swelling, nausea, redness, elevated skin temperature, and white drainage from the incision. Upon observation, the PT believes the patient has an infection and calls the physician. The PT should document the events that took place, the observations, any assessments, and his or her response. Documenting response to treatment and your actions when appropriate helps to show patient management and clinical decision making in response to positive or negative events.

PROVIDE PROOF THAT CARE IS "REASONABLE AND NECESSARY"

Our documentation must provide evidence that physical therapy services are reasonable and necessary. The Centers for Medicare & Medicaid Services (CMS) has set forth criteria that need to be met for services to be considered reasonable and necessary. These criteria include the following[8(p168-172)]:

- The services shall be considered under accepted standards of medical practice to be a specific and effective treatment for the patient's condition.
- The services provided to the patient are at a level of complexity and sophistication that can only be provided by a therapist or assistant under appropriate supervision.
- The condition of the patient is such that services can only safely and effectively be provided only by a therapist or assistant under appropriate supervision.
- Though the patient's medical condition is an important factor in considering whether or not services are skilled, a beneficiary's diagnosis or prognosis should never be the sole factor in deciding that a service is or is not skilled.
- An expectation that the patient's condition will improve significantly in a reasonable (and generally predictable) period of time or that the services must be necessary for the establishment of a safe and effective maintenance program required in connection with a specific disease state. In the case of a progressive degenerative disease, service may be necessary to determine the need for assistive or adaptive equipment and/or to establish a program to maximize patient function.
- The amount, frequency, and duration of the services must be reasonable under accepted standards of practice in the local area or according to state or national therapy associations.

The deciding factors are always whether the services are considered reasonable, effective treatments for the patient's condition, and require the skills of a therapist (skilled care, see next section) or whether they can be safely and effectively carried out by nonskilled personnel without the supervision of qualified professionals.[8]

Documentation to justify reasonable and necessary services includes initial documentation that demonstrates a relationship between the patient's pathology, the identified impairments, activity limitations, and participation restrictions. The documentation includes a description of how the impairments have led to limitations in a patient's activity level or restrictions in a patient's ability to participate in normal life roles or tasks. Documentation outlines a specific plan of care to address these limitations and includes ongoing reassessments, including objective functional measures. The documentation must convey how the interventions will influence the patient's condition. Furthermore, the documentation must show how the interventions provided included the unique and complex skills or decision making of a therapist.

In most cases, the PT proves that services are reasonable and necessary in the initial documentation; nevertheless, it is important for a PTA to recognize when the intervention is no longer reasonable or necessary. Intervention may no longer be medically necessary if (1) the patient has met all the goals that have been established by the physical therapist, (2) the patient is no longer benefiting from the intervention, or (3) the services can be carried out through home exercise instructions or by untrained personnel. Treatment might also exceed criteria for medical necessity if the patient, family, or caregiver(s) has unrealistic expectations for recovery.[9] Documentation showing objective, comparative data can help provide evidence that a patient is progressing toward the goals stated in the plan of care. Documentation can then further support the need for subsequent or continued interventions due to medical necessity or it can provide a rationale for discontinuing physical therapy services.

SKILLED CARE

Skilled, rehabilitative therapy occurs when the skills of a therapist are necessary to safely and effectively furnish a recognized therapy service whose goal is improvement of an impairment or functional limitation.[8] In order for a physical therapy intervention to be considered skilled, a patient must have a pathology or injury that results in a documented physical or functional limitation and requires a sophisticated and complex intervention that can only be carried out by a licensed PT or a PTA under the supervision of a PT. This intervention requires the unique judgment and skill of a trained individual for both safety and effectiveness. Skilled interventions have been proven safe, effective, and specific to the patient's condition. Services that are not considered skilled care are often known as *maintenance therapy*. Maintenance therapy services can be provided by a nonlicensed individual, such as a family member or caregiver who has had some training from a skilled professional, or by the patient through independent home exercises. Maintenance services are not reimbursed by Medicare or many other third-party payers.[10] Documentation must describe how the interventions provided included the unique and complex skills or decision making of a therapist. Clinicians can further justify skilled services by describing the actual skills provided or decision making that was implemented for a particular patient treatment (ie, provided facilitation to the wrist/finger extensors to improve the patient's ability to position her hand for grasp).

DEMONSTRATE THE CLINICAL DECISION-MAKING PROCESS

From initial examination to discharge, physical therapy documentation should provide a picture of the clinician's decision-making process and clinical judgment.[2,9,11] Documentation that demonstrates clinical decision making also improves the provider's credibility with third-party payers.[5] An individual who does not know the patient should be able to read the physical therapy records and identify a logical, stepwise progression from initial examination to discharge. Lewis indicated that "documentation of all elements of the patient/client management model ... should harmonize."[2(p30)] Documentation should reflect logical decisions and sound judgment by showing direct links between subjective remarks, patient impairments and functional problems, goals, interventions, changes in interventions, and rationale for discharge.

Both the PT and PTA have specific roles in making sure that this occurs:

- Data collected during the initial examination should be reflected in the plan of care. For example, goals written by the PT should reflect impairments (ie, decreased range of motion, decreased strength), activity limitations (ie, difficulty transferring, decreased independence with gait), and participation restrictions (ie, unable to work) identified during the initial examination (PT role).
- The plan of care should include physical therapy interventions that are aimed at reducing the identified impairments, activity limitations, and participation restrictions (PT role).
- Changes in patient status should prompt changes in the plan of care (PT and PTA role to recognize and record changes in patient status, PTA role to communicate changes to the PT, PT role to adjust the plan of care based on patient changes).

As a PTA, you can further contribute to the decision-making process by collecting pertinent subjective and objective patient data following the initial examination.

Subjective data often gathered and recorded by a PTA include the following:

- Asking the patient about his or her response to a previous treatment.
- Inquiring about compliance with a home exercise program.
- Asking the patient whether the treatment has improved function.

When asking a patient whether the treatment has improved function, it is important to refer back to the initial documentation to see what limitations the patient had when he or she started the episode of care. That way, you can be specific in your inquiries.

Prior to collecting objective data through tests and measurements, it is important to see what measurements were taken during the initial evaluation. That way, you have a baseline to which your measurements can be compared. In addition, it is important to try to speak with the PT about the patient prior to the treatment session. At that time you can ask whether or not additional tests and measurements are needed.

Objective data often gathered by a PTA include the following:

- Goniometric measurements
- Manual muscle testing
- Functional status (bed mobility, transfers, gait)

The PTA should record subjective patient comments and results of relevant tests and measurements in interim notes or daily notes. These notes serve to reveal changes in impairments, activity limitations, and participation restrictions that were found during the initial examination. Findings that warrant a re-evaluation, changes in the plan of care, or discharge should also be provided in the documentation by the PTA and communicated to the PT.

When there is consistency between the initial examination and subsequent notes, the clinical decision-making process is more easily identified. Ongoing documentation of subjective remarks and objective findings tells the story of the patient's response to therapy. In addition, consistency between initial and subsequent documentation makes it easier for the clinician(s) to identify progress or lack thereof. This also allows the PT to easily update goals and interventions as needed. This process will be described in more detail in Chapter 4.

REFERENCES

1. Inaba M, Jones SL. Medical documentation for third-party payers. *Phys Ther.* 1977;57:791–794.
2. Lewis DK. Do the write thing: document everything. *PT Magazine.* 2002;10(7):30–34.
3. American Physical Therapy Association House of Delegates. *Standards of Ethical Conduct for the Physical Therapist Assistant.* HOD 06-09-20-18. Available at: http://www.apta.org/uploadedFiles/APTAorg/About_Us/Policies/HOD/Ethics/Standards.pdf. Accessed May 18, 2011.
4. Hebert LA. Basics of Medicare documentation for physical therapy. *Clinical Management in Physical Therapy.* 1981;1(3):13–14.
5. Baeten AM. Documentation: the reviewer perspective. *Top Geriatr Rehabil.* 1997;13(1):14–22.
6. American Physical Therapy Association. *The Guide to Physical Therapist Practice.* Alexandria, Va: American Physical Therapy Association; 2001. Available at: guidetoptpractice.apta.org. Accessed February 18, 2012.
7. Goode N. The reliable resource: physical therapy documentation. *PT Magazine.* 1999;7(9):30–31.
8. Centers for Medicare and Medicaid Services. Pub. No. 100-02 Medicare Benefit Policy Manual, Chapter 15-Section 220. Available at: http://www.cms.gov/Manuals/IOM/ItemDetail.asp?ItemID=CMS012673. Published 2006. Accessed February 3, 2012.
9. Redgate N, Foto M. Pay by the rules: avoid Medicare audits and reduce payment denials with a sound strategy and proper documentation. *Physical Therapy Products.* October/November 2003:28–30.
10. Moorhead JF, Clifford J. Determining medical necessity of outpatient physical therapy services. *Am J Med Qual.* 1992;7(3):81–84.
11. Arriaga R. Liability awareness. Stories from the front: documentation and clinical decision making: a real-life scenario illustrates some basic risk-management principles. *PT Magazine.* 2002;10(5):46–49.

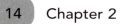

REVIEW QUESTIONS

1. List reasons for documenting.

2. What are examples of subjective and objective data that can be gathered by a PTA?

3. How can a clinician integrate the clinical decision-making process in his or her documentation?

4. Give some examples of how a PTA can assist in showing clinical decision making.

5. What are the criteria for determining whether a treatment or intervention is reasonable and necessary?

6. Who determines medical necessity initially?

7. What is the difference between skilled care and maintenance therapy? Provide an example of each.

8. What is the role of the PTA in determining medical necessity?

9. How does the patient's rehabilitation potential influence his or her need for medically necessary skilled care?

10. Review the *Standards of Ethical Conduct for the Physical Therapist Assistant*[3] (http://www.apta.org/Core Documents) and identify your professional obligation(s) that pertain to documentation.

APPLICATION EXERCISES

I. Read through the following examination/evaluation and answer the questions that follow.

Date: March 15, 2004

Pr: 27 y.o. s/p (L) wrist and ankle fx; <u>Referral</u>: Begin gentle wrist and ankle AROM & PROM; May begin using crutches with platform for (L) UE. PWB 50% on (L) LE.

S: *HPI*: 4 weeks s/p fall (~25') from a logging truck landing on his (L) side (2/1/04). Pt. sustained fx of the (L) distal radius and ulna and (L) distal tibia and fibula. Pt. underwent ORIF for the wrist and ankle immediately after the injury. He was placed in a short-arm cast for the UE and short-leg cast for the LE. He was NWB on the (L) LE initially and has been unable to use crutches due to not being allowed to bear weight on the affected UE. At the time of the fall, the pt. also sustained a mild concussion. He was hospitalized for 5 days following the injury. While hospitalized he received PT to learn how to negotiate his w/c and perform transfers. Both casts were removed yesterday and his ankle was placed in a removable splint. He reports taking ibuprofen PRN for pain.

C/C: Pain and stiffness in (L) UE & LE with decreased functional use of (B). Doesn't like using w/c for mobility. Unable to work. Requiring assist with self-care activities and home management.

Living situation: Right-hand dominant; Lives with wife and 2 small children in single-level home with 2 steps @ entrance and hand rail on the (R). Prior to injury pt. was employed as a construction worker and independent in all functional activities in and around the home. He has been off work since the injury. Pt. is unable to drive and is relying on his wife & mother for transportation. No significant PMH or history of fracture. Reports being a nonsmoker and nondrinker. Family history is (+) for OA.

Pt's Goals: Return to previous level of function and RTW ASAP. Learn to ambulate with crutches.

O: *AROM*: (R) UE & LE WNL; (L) shoulder, elbow, & hip WNL.

		AROM	PROM
(L) wrist:	Flexion	20°	25°
	Extension	10°	15°
	UD	10°	15°
	RD	15°	15°
	Supination	30°	35°
	Pronation	40°	45°
(L) hand:	Pt. can perform a full fist but it is difficult 2° to edema. Thumb IP, MCP, and CMC AROM is WNL		
(L) knee:		0–100°	0–110°
(L) ankle:	DF	–10°	–5°
	PF	20°	25°
	Inv	5°	5°
	Ev	0°	5°

Strength: (R) UE & LE 5/5; (L) shoulder and hip 4/5; (L) elbow, wrist, knee, & ankle deferred 2° to acuity.

Girth: wrist figure 8 (R): 36 cm (L): 37.2 cm; ankle figure 8 (R): 42 cm (L): 44.1 cm.

Sensation: (L) wrist and ankle intact to light touch & (=) when compared to (R).

Circulation: 2+ at radial & dorsal pedal arteries on the (L).

Special Tests: N/A @ this time 2° to acuity.

Gait: Amb. 50' PWB 50% (L) LE using crutches with (L) UE platform using step to gait pattern with CGAx1 for sequencing and balance.

Transfers: (I) bed to and from chair, chair to and from toilet, sit to and from stand; all PWB on (L) LE.

Bed Mobility: (I) all areas.

Tx & HEP: AROM & PROM for (L) wrist for flexion, extension, pronation, & supination and for (L) ankle DF and PF, used opposite foot for self PROM of ankle; performed AROM for all digits and thumb; initiated compression glove for edema to be worn at night; instructed pt. in elevation and compression wrapping for ankle and wrist; instructed pt. in use of crutches The pt. performed all ex. x20 reps (I) and verbalized understanding of all precautions.

A: 27 y.o. RHD male 4 wks s/p fall where he sustained fx to the (L) wrist & ankle. Now decreased AROM, PROM, strength, and weight bearing restrictions are causing inability to ambulate, perform self-care, drive, or perform home management tasks without assistance. He is also unable to work @ this time. Skilled services necessary to instruct pt. in safe, appropriate ROM ex. and progression, use of assistive device & gait training as ordered. Pt. will also require instruction in strengthening ex. and retraining in functional mobility to prepare for return to normal lifestyle and RTW. Pt. able to communicate without limitations and demonstrates excellent motivation and good potential for full recovery. No comorbidities identified that could affect outcome at this time.

Anticipated Goals and Expected Outcomes:

At the end of 2 weeks, the pt. will:

1.   Increase AROM 10–15° for the wrist, forearm, and ankle to improve use of UE and LE during functional activities.
2.   Decrease edema by 0.5 cm for the wrist and ankle.
3.   Ambulate 200′ with crutches with (L) UE platform PWB 50% on (L) LE independently.
4.   Perform all self-care independently.
5.   Perform a full fist without limitations.

At the end of 16 weeks (time of d/c), the pt. will:

1.   Achieve AROM of the wrist, forearm, and ankle 90–100% of opposite to allow use during basic care, home tasks, and work activities.
2.   Achieve grip and pinch strength 80% of (R) to allow use during basic care, home tasks, and work activities.
3.   Be independent with all self-care & home management tasks.
4.   Ambulate independently on all surfaces without use of assistive device.
5.   Ascend and descend a flight of stairs independently without assistive device.
6.   Drive without restrictions.
7.   RTW @ previous level of employment.

P: See pt. 3x/wk for next 3–4 mos. to work on AROM & PROM of the wrist and ankle; LE ex. for the hip, knee, shoulder, and elbow; gait training; functional mobility & strengthening to involved joints when appropriate. Will progress pt. as tolerated when appropriate & according to MD orders. Pt. is in agreement with the above stated plan.

John Smith, PT

1.   List 5 of the patient's impairments.

2.   List 5 of the patient's functional (activity) limitations and participation restrictions.

3.   Is this patient disabled? Why or why not?

4.   In this example, how are the patient's impairments creating functional limitations and disability?

5.   List 5 pieces of subjective data found in the evaluation.

6.   List 5 pieces of objective data found in the evaluation.

7.   How did the PT describe the need for skilled care?

8.   What information would you need to provide in a progress note for this patient to show medical necessity and the need for further skilled care?

9. Is this patient's care medically necessary? Why or why not? What evidence is there of medical necessity?

10. What other providers/individuals might be interested in looking at this patient's note(s)?

II. Read through the following scenarios and decide whether the treatment would be considered *maintenance* or *skilled*. Give an explanation for your answer. If you choose maintenance, what are some things that you should do (as a PTA) to discontinue treatment?

1. You are working with a patient in a nursing home who has severe Alzheimer's disease. Every afternoon, you take her for a walk through the hallways around the building. She demonstrates weakness in her right ankle, and there is a foot slap during the contact phase of gait. She can control it if given verbal cuing. You have been working with her for a month. You are not seeing any follow-through from one session to the next, and she has not progressed her distance or level of assistance in the last 2 weeks.

2. You have been working for a home health agency in the evenings to make some extra money. The patient you are currently seeing has not shown improvement in the 2 weeks. She is an 85-year-old woman with Parkinson's disease who lives with her daughter. You are considering recommending discharge when one day the patient's daughter tells you that her mother enjoys having you come in, and they really believe that you are helping. You think the patient's daughter could carry out the program independently.

3. You are working in a skilled nursing unit and you are assigned a patient who requires maximum assist for transfers and cannot participate in therapy due to lethargy and confusion. Every day you do PROM to all extremities and transfer the patient to the bedside chair.

4. You and your supervising PT are working in an outpatient physical therapy clinic with a patient who has a frozen shoulder. She has been participating in therapy for about 6 weeks. During that time she has made a substantial amount of progress. Recently her ROM has started to plateau. The patient attends therapy twice a week for stretching and joint mobilizations.

5. You are working on gait training with a patient who had a right cerebrovascular accident (CVA) and has resultant left hemiplegia. While ambulating, you provide tactile and verbal cuing to the quadriceps to achieve full knee extension in late swing. The patient can respond to your cues about 50% of the time. Gait has improved over the last week as evidenced by decreased level of assistance provided by the therapist.

III. Interview a PT or PTA who has been practicing in the field for more than 10 years. Ask him or her how documentation requirements have changed. Also, discuss why he or she thinks that documentation is important.

Chapter 3

Documentation Formats

Mia L. Erickson, PT, EdD, CHT, ATC

CHAPTER OBJECTIVES

After reading this chapter, the student will be able to do the following:

1. List 4 types of documentation formats used in physical therapy.
2. Examine different types of physical therapy documentation formats.
3. Describe each type of documentation.
4. Explain advantages and disadvantages of different documentation formats including the narrative, problem-oriented medical record (POMR), subjective–objective–assessment–plan (SOAP) notes, and functional outcomes reporting (FOR).
5. Differentiate between information found in the S, O, A, and P portions of a SOAP note.
6. Identify positive and negative aspects of using forms and templates.
7. Identify positive and negative aspects of computerized documentation.

Documentation in physical therapy practice can take on a variety of formats depending on the type of patients being treated, practice setting or type of facility, state laws and practice acts, and reimbursement requirements. Documentation formats include narrative reports, the POMR, SOAP notes, and the FOR (Figure 3-1). A brief discussion of each of these formats is provided in this chapter.

NARRATIVE

In narrative documentation, the clinician describes the patient encounter written mainly in paragraph format.

Several problems with the narrative record have been reported. First, narrative notes may lack structure, making the writer prone to omit important details. In addition, there is a high degree of note-writing variability among clinicians.[1] When medical notes lack structure and vary between clinicians, it becomes very difficult to read and locate necessary information. For example, it would be very time consuming for a physician or case manager to sort through a chart filled with unstructured narrative entries to locate information regarding the patient's ability to transfer or ambulate. Furthermore, following the clinician's problem-solving process can be difficult in narrative reports.[2]

Nevertheless, the use of narrative notes still occurs, and ways to improve readability with this format have been suggested. First, when using the narrative format, Quinn and Gordon[1] recommended developing an outline of information to cover so that important details are not omitted. Also, using headings can make information easier to find. Headings used in the narrative format are at the discretion of the clinician writing the note and may or may not be used.

Narrative Example 1

Date: 3/3/04

Patient: John Smith

Pt. RTC reporting no adverse effects from treatment last visit or from HEP. He stated that he feels as though his wrist & ankle are moving a little better and the edema in the hand has decreased. He reports that he is able to shower (I) using a plastic chair in the tub and feels like he has improved with his ability to dress himself. AROM of the (L) wrist is as follows: flexion 30°, extension 30°, UD 15°, RD 20°, supination 45°, and pronation 60°; (L) knee: 0–135°; (L) ankle

Erickson M, McKnight R. *Documentation Basics: A Guide for the Physical Therapist Assistant, Second Edition* (pp. 19-32)
© 2012 SLACK Incorporated

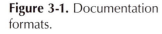

Figure 3-1. Documentation formats.

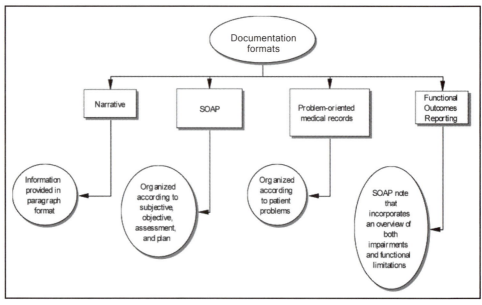

DF-PF 5–45°. Figure 8 wrist girth is 35.5 cm and ankle figure 8 girth is 43 cm on the (L). Pt. is ambulating household distances (I) with crutches using (L) UE platform, PWB 50% on the (L) LE. He notes (I) with all transfers and self-care. Tx consisted of gentle AROM and PROM for 30' to the (L) wrist and forearm in the directions of flexion, extension, supination, & pronation and to the (L) ankle for DF, PF, inv, & ev. Pt. also performed AROM for the hand. The pt. has made improvements in AROM and has decreased edema. Improvements have allowed pt. to improve his ability to ambulate (I) and perform self-care. Will continue to have the pt. perform his HEP and RTC on 3/5/04.

    Bill Jones, PTA

There are times when the narrative format is the most appropriate format to use. These include describing a sequence of events, brief interactions with patients, conversations with other health care providers, or any other situation that requires a detailed explanation and no other documentation formats are appropriate. In these instances, you can simply describe the situation and how it affects the patient in a brief paragraph or narrative note. Narrative notes are sometimes the easiest to use when you just need to describe the details of a situation and you are trying to paint a vivid description of what happened.

Narrative Example 2

    Date: 6/18/03
    Patient: John Smith
    Spoke with patient's physician today regarding the amount of weight bearing he is allowed to perform when ambulating with the platform crutches. He stated that his fx sites on the radius and ulna are stable and healing well, and he can WBAT on the UE. Will report conversation to the

PT and have patient continue to use crutches with platform on the (L), allowing him to weight bear through the UE as instructed by the physician.

    Bill Jones, PTA

PROBLEM-ORIENTED MEDICAL RECORD

The POMR was introduced by Lawrence Weed to provide medical students with a structured documentation format oriented around the patient's problems.[2] He believed that the narrative format was often confusing and unorganized, making it difficult to determine how the physician defined and treated various patient problems.[2] The POMR became a type of documentation used mainly by physicians.

In the POMR, the first page of the medical record consisted of a patient problem list. This served as the table of contents for the remainder of the medical record.

POMR Example 1

    Patient: John Smith
    Problem 1: Decreased A/PROM left wrist
    Problem 2: Decreased A/PROM left ankle
    Problem 3: Decreased strength left wrist
    Problem 4: Decreased strength left ankle
    Problem 5: Decreases (I) with ambulation and functional activities

Subsequent entries, or progress notes, were organized according to each problem. The physician discussed management of each problem in separate entries using the following headings:

- Subjective data: Symptomatic data provided by the patient.

- Objective data: Results of tests and measurements performed or physical exam data.
- Impression (Imp.): The practitioner's impression of the patient and that particular problem.
- Treatment and therapy (Rx): Treatment or therapy provided for that particular problem on that day or during that session.
- Immediate plans (Plan): Treatment plan for that particular problem.

POMR Example 2

Date: 3/3/04
Patient: John Smith
Problem #1: Decreased A/PROM left wrist.
Subj: Pt. reports no adverse effects from last treatment; states that the wrist and hand are moving better and edema has decreased.
Obj: AROM (L) wrist: flexion 30°, extension 30°, UD 15°, RD 20°, supination 45°, and pronation 60°.
Imp: A/PROM improving with exercise.
Rx: 2 x 10 reps AROM and PROM for flexion, extension, supination, and pronation.
Plan: Have pt. continue with HEP and RTC in 2 days for progression of exercise.

Using this format, the reader can identify the patient's care for each of the identified problems.

Major advantages of the POMR include the following[3-8]:

- Provides organization and structure to the medical information.
- Includes a comprehensive list of the patient's problems.
- Discusses each of the patient's problems separately.
- Provides a specific plan for managing each of the patient's problems (ie, treatment is problem oriented).
- Allows a physician who is interested in a particular problem to go directly to that aspect of the note, thus improving communication among care providers.
- Provides a chronological sequence of interventions for a particular problem, better outlining the problem-solving process.

Regardless of the benefits provided with the POMR, authors have reported problems with it as well. First, the POMR separates, or fragments, patients according to their problems, and this might pose a problem in complex cases if a provider does not see the "whole patient."[7] In the case of John Smith, it is possible that a therapist working with the upper extremity might not be aware of the lower extremity problems without reading separate chart entries. This could be very time consuming. In addition, for patients with multiple problems, the POMR can become increasingly complex, requiring an extraordinary amount of time for an individual who is managing multiple problems. In our example, the patient has many problems,

and for one therapist, this could result in as many as 5 to 6 different chart entries per visit. Therefore, it has typically not been suitable for more complex rehabilitation patients.[3]

More contemporary versions of the POMR have emerged that are centered around patient problems. They often include the problem, associated goal, current status, and treatment directed at the problem. They may or may not include SOAP elements.[1] Now, however, they are usually included in a single chart entry or template (Figure 3-2).

SOAP NOTES

The SOAP note evolved from the POMR documentation format initially provided by Weed[2] as described in the preceding section. As with the POMR, S, or subjective, should include anything the patient tells you pertaining to his or her injuries or problems. Subjective information can also be any information provided by the patient's family or caregivers. The O, or objective, section should include relevant tests and measurements performed, the patient's functional status, and physical therapy interventions provided for that day of service. The interventions include procedural interventions, like exercise and modalities, but should also include any collaboration with other disciplines and patient or family education provided. Unlike the POMR, in the SOAP format, the physical therapy interventions are written in the objective portion of the note. The interpretation, or impression, has been designated A for assessment. In SOAP format, the P stands for plan. More detailed examples of information provided in the S, O, A, and P portions of the notes can be found in Figures 3-3 through 3-6.

Unlike the POMR, one SOAP note generally includes information pertaining to all of the patient's problems. Occasionally, the entire SOAP note is preceded by a problem (Pr) section. The Pr section contains information pertaining to the medical diagnosis, referral information (see SOAP below), or information taken from the medical record. You will read more about the SOAP sections, including the Pr section, in Chapter 7.

The SOAP format is now widely used by a variety of medical and rehabilitation professionals, although it is no longer associated with the POMR.[1] SOAP has become a stand-alone format for documentation. Like the POMR, SOAP note documentation provides structure to medical record entries and should be used to show logical decision making by using subjective and objective information to determine an assessment and plan.

SOAP Example

(Please note: This is the same information that was provided in the narrative and POMR notes above. Pay particular attention to the organization of subjective and

Name: James Wilson
Date of service: 2/1/2012
Medical Dx: 70 y.o. male; 2 weeks s/p hip fracture

Problem:	Associated goal:	Current status:	Treatment provided to meet goal:
1. Pt. is unable to ascend and descend 1 flight of stairs in his home without assistance	Ascend and descend a flight of stairs (I) without assistive device	Pt. can ascend and descend 3 stairs PWB 50% (L) LE with a handrail and straight cane with CGA x 1	15' hip, quadriceps and hamstring strengthening, A/PROM (L) ankle, knee, and hip, and 15' stairs training
2. Pt. is unable to ambulate necessary distance and velocity for community ambulation	The pt. will ambulate 500-100' with straight cane (I) at a velocity of 1.2 m/sec or better	The pt. ambulates 150' with constant supervision due to balance deficits with a standard walker PWB 50% (L) LE	15' gait training and 15' balance training using limits of stability and visual cues

Total treatment time=60'

S: Pt. reports that he is doing well and feels like his gait is improving

Overall Impression: The pt. has progressed in his ability to negotiate stairs, now performing with CGA opposed to min (A) x 1 at initial evaluation. Gait has also improved in that he is no longer requiring cues for limited weight-bearing and he is able to self-correct balance ~50% of the time

Plan: Continue with these two primary goals, progress his balance program as his weight-bearing status improves.

Signature:

Figure 3-2. More contemporary version of POMR.

objective information as well as the assessment and plan under the appropriate headings)

Date: 3/3/04

Patient: John Smith

Pr: 27 y.o. s/p (L) wrist and ankle fx; Referral: Begin gentle wrist and ankle AROM & PROM.

S: Pt. RTC reporting no adverse effects from treatment last visit or from HEP. He stated that his wrist & ankle are moving a little better and the edema in the hand has decreased. He reports that he is able to shower (I) using a plastic chair in the tub and feels like he has improved c̄ his ability to dress himself.

O: AROM: (L) wrist: flexion 30°, extension 30°, UD 15°, RD 20°, supination 45°, pronation 60°; (L) knee: 0–135°; (L) ankle: DF 5°, PF 45°. Girth: (L) wrist figure 8: 35.5 cm and (L) ankle figure 8: 43 cm. Tx: gentle AROM and PROM for 30' to the (L) wrist & forearm for flexion, extension, supination, & pronation. Pt. also performed hand AROM.

A: The pt. has made improvements in AROM and has shown decreased edema. Improvements in AROM have allowed pt. to improve ability to ambulate (I) and perform self-care.

P: Will continue to have the pt. perform his HEP and RTC on 3/5/04 for further exercise progression.

Bill Jones, PTA

Even though SOAP notes provide a consistent and concise format for documenting the patient's subjective remarks, objective exam findings, interventions, the provider's overall impression, and the overall treatment plan, the documentation format has been scrutinized. Several reasons for this exist. First, objective findings are often written in terms of impairments, such as range of motion, strength, balance, etc. Furthermore, links between impairments and function and between improvements in impairments and improved functional capabilities are usually implied rather than described in detail.[9,10] These problems often result

Figure 3-3. Subjective.

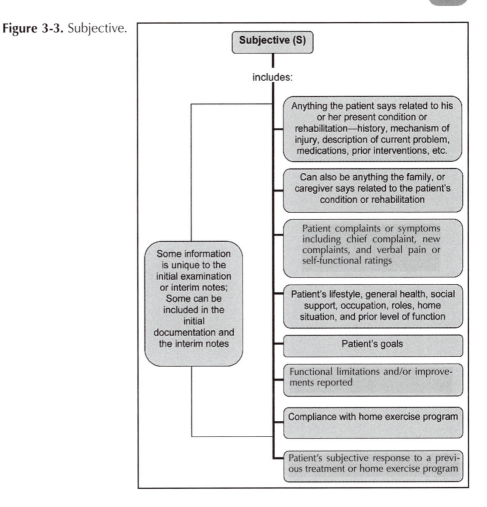

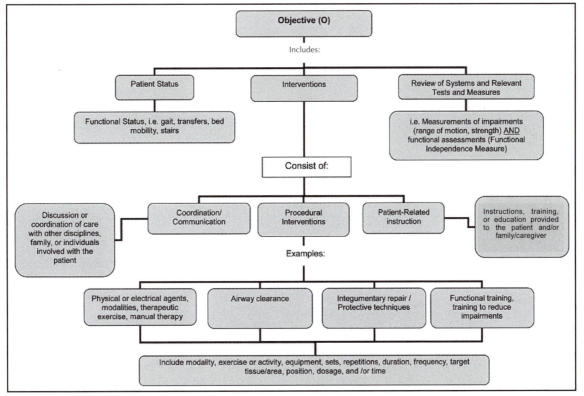

Figure 3-4. Objective.

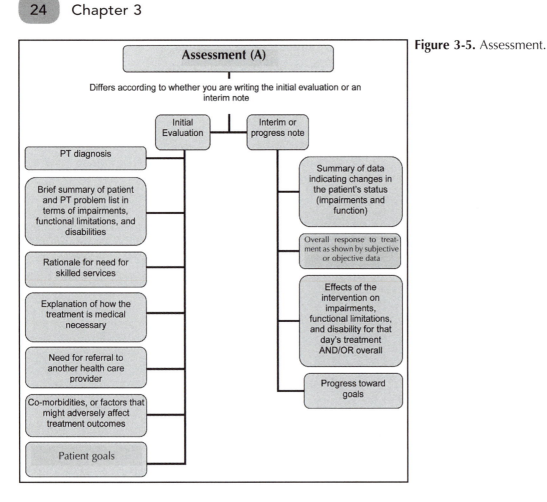

Figure 3-5. Assessment.

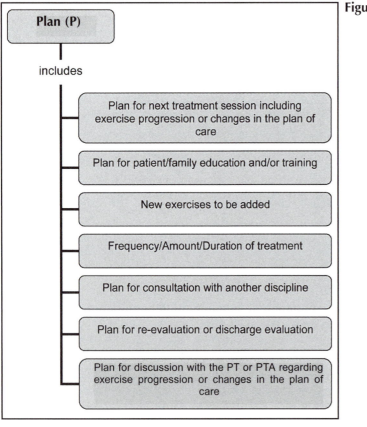

Figure 3-6. Plan.

in documentation centered around the patient's complaints and impairments, rather than functional changes. In addition, SOAP notes usually do not describe how the interventions are contributing to improving impairments or function. Nevertheless, the SOAP format is widely accepted and can be an appropriate form of documentation if its emphasis shifts away from complaints and impairments toward *linking impairment, function, and intervention.*

FUNCTIONAL OUTCOMES REPORTING

Functional outcomes reporting is becoming more popular in rehabilitation. This type of documentation has an increased focus on patient function.[1] Advantages of FOR have been identified. FOR clearly lays out the relationship between the patient's impairments and the ability to perform functional tasks, and it improves readability for non-health care providers reviewing documentation.[1,11] Authors have recommended integrating this approach into the SOAP structure described above.[1,11] The integration of SOAP and FOR can be done by making the following additions to SOAP:

- Objective (O) section: Clearly and objectively describe the patient's functional status, including functional activities that are specific to that patient, in addition to documenting impairments.[11]
- Assessment (A) section: (a) List only those impairments being addressed with therapy; (b) describes how improvement in impairments will lead to improvement in function, including both activities and participation; (c) provides complicating factors; that is, comorbidities; and (d) PTs write goals using functional terminology.[11]
- Include the functional goal(s) at the top of daily and progress notes that were emphasized during that day of treatment.[1]

FOR/SOAP Example

(Please note: The following is the same example that was used to demonstrate narrative, POMR, and SOAP formats. This example combines the FOR with the SOAP format as recommended by Abeln.[11] Additions are presented in italics):

Date: 3/3/04

Patient: John Smith

Goals: (1) Increase AROM in the hand, wrist, and forearm to allow (I) with ADLs, work activities, and child care. (2) Increase ankle AROM to allow normal gait pattern.

S: Pt. RTC reporting no adverse effects from treatment last visit or from HEP. He stated that his wrist & ankle are moving a little better and the edema in the hand has decreased. He reports that he is able to shower (I) using a plastic chair in the tub and feels like he has improved c̄ his ability to dress himself.

O: AROM: (L) wrist: flexion 30°, extension 30°, UD 15°, RD 20°, supination 45°, pronation 60°; (L) knee: 0–135°; (L) ankle: DF 5°, PF 45°. Girth: (L) wrist figure 8: 35.5 cm and (L) ankle figure 8: 43 cm. *Functional Status: Gait: Ambulates household distances with (B) axillary crutches with (L) UE platform, PWB 50% (L), (I). Transfers: (I) with all transfers. Self-care: (I) with showering and dressing. IADLs: Unable to work; Unable to assist wife with child care duties.* Tx: gentle AROM and PROM for 30" to the (L) wrist & forearm for flexion, extension, supination, & pronation and for the (L) ankle for PF, DF, inversion and eversion. Pt. also performed hand AROM.

A: The pt. has made improvements in AROM and has decreased edema, although both continue to be impairments. *Decreased edema and exercise have improved AROM allowing improved use of wrist & hand during self-care and use of ankle for normal gait pattern. Continues to require use of crutches 2° to PWB status—this is limiting his ability to ambulate without an assistive device.*

P: Will continue to have the pt. perform his HEP and return on 3/5/04 for appropriate ex. progression.

Bill Jones, PTA

This chapter outlines several different types of physical therapy notes, each being used to document patient care. These included the narrative note, POMR, SOAP notes, and FOR. In hospitals and clinical settings, you are likely to encounter a wide variety of documentation formats, and it is important that you adhere to both state and federal laws as well as your facility's approved format. It is the author's experience that the SOAP format is most widely used; however, the POMR done in a single note is becoming increasingly more popular in this contemporary format. Also, the blending of SOAP and FOR is becoming more common. Narrative notes also serve distinct purposes as previously described. Although there is no evidence suggesting superiority of one type of note over another, you will soon find that in real-world clinical practice, you are likely to apply principles from all documentation formats, thus using a combination of narrative, POMR, SOAP, and FOR. The authors of this text have selected the SOAP format to provide a framework for teaching basic documentation skills. This format was selected because of its prevalence in clinical practice and because of its adaptability to a variety of documentation styles, including electronic documentation. Thus, once you have learned the SOAP format, you will be able to adapt your note writing to meet employer and payer expectations. While the SOAP format will serve as the basic structure for your notes, additional emphasis will be placed on documenting the patient's functional status; linking impairments, function, and interventions; linking interventions with improvement; referring to the initial evaluative note; demonstrating clinical decision making; and integrating medical necessity and need for skilled care.

TEMPLATES AND FILL-IN FORMS

In order to facilitate documentation and eliminate time constraints, clinicians often use a variety of documentation templates and fill-in forms. Forms can be either paper or computer based. These forms not only save time but have potential to minimize writing, improve accuracy and consistency across patients, prompt clinicians to provide necessary data,[12] and include essential documentation requirements set forth by Medicare or other third-party payers.[13] Initial evaluations, daily and progress notes, re-evaluations, discharge summaries, and physician progress updates can be written using standard forms developed by individual facilities. Several paper examples of standardized forms and templates have been provided in Appendix B. *The Guide to Physical Therapist Practice*[14] and "Defensible Documentation"[15] also include documentation templates for use in physical therapy practice.

Forms and templates can also provide a mechanism for multidisciplinary documentation in which each discipline has its own section to complete on the same form. For example, in inpatient rehabilitation settings and in skilled nursing facilities, Medicare payment is determined by data provided through multidisciplinary fill-in forms. An example of a multidisciplinary form is the Minimum Data Set,[18] used in skilled nursing facilities.

Though fill-in forms and templates often ease time constraints and improve consistency, both PTs and PTAs must take care to not allow the form to "dictate" the session. This is especially important for students and new graduates, who may feel that they cannot deviate from the form. In some instances, clinical instructors and employers will require students and new graduates to document using one of the above-described formats (narrative, SOAP, etc) rather than using the standard facility templates or fill-in forms. More important, forms can promote incomplete documentation.[16,17] Providers must be sure that forms used not only contain all essential information but also have areas where you are able to add narrative comments.[16] These areas allow you to describe aspects of the patient's care that are not part of the standard template or form. Remember to document all relevant aspects of the patient's care, including characteristics unique to some patients that might not be part of the standard templates or forms. Another problem with templates is that they are often geared toward the patient population treated most at the facility. It might be difficult to use these forms when documenting on patients with less common diagnoses. Several documentation templates can be found in Appendix B.

THE ELECTRONIC MEDICAL RECORD

Computer-based documentation, or the electronic medical record (EMR), is one of the most rapidly growing areas for the use of computer technology in rehabilitation.[19] The EMR can range from basic word processing documents with fill-in form features to complex computerized documentation software packages that link to a clinic's billing and scheduling software. Initial examination/evaluations, daily and progress notes, re-evaluations, and discharge summaries are most often integrated into the EMR for PTs. These often consist of commonly used templates based around body systems or regions that standardize terminology and incorporate check boxes, pull-down menus, and other time-saving efforts (Figure 3-7). Some software packages can generate notes to the physician or case manager populated by previously recorded patient data. Additional benefits to computerized documentation packages include more timely submission of bills and records to payers, improved readability, eased ability to build databases for research, and improved visit and insurance tracking. Another added benefit includes the incorporation of customizable templates based on clinic demand or need.

However, there are several important considerations for using the EMR. First is the cost–benefit ratio. The benefits of using the software must offset its expense. In addition, staff training, technical support, rapid obsolescence of hardware and software, upgrade costs, and daily work flow are important considerations for implementing an EMR. Computerized systems do not always save time, and templates that accompany software packages may not accommodate all patient types seen in a particular facility. There should be some sort of template customization allowed to increase the documentation flexibility between patient types.[19] There are times when the complex patient's case does not fit easily into the computerized templates and clinicians must type the majority of the note in free text boxes. Also, it is difficult to capture medical necessity and the need for skilled care in a set of check boxes due to the individual differences between patients, and this may need to be free texted as well because it is such an important component of the documentation. The need to free text a lot of information quickly decreases the efficiency. It is also important that clinicians do not get into a routine of documenting the same things for every patient; computerized software generates standard phrases, and notes can quickly start appearing the same for each patient.

Furthermore, the clinic must be prepared for regularly scheduled system backups, upgrades, and maintenance of main and individual computer terminals so that critical information is not lost. There must also be processes for storing system backup files. Abeln[17] suggested storing backups away from the computer systems themselves. Finally, there must be a mechanism to record, give reason for, and authenticate late entries.[17]

Types of computerized documentation packages include the following:

- Clinicient (http://www.clinicient.com)
- TurboPT (www.gssinc.com)
- ReDoc (www.rehabdocumentation.com)

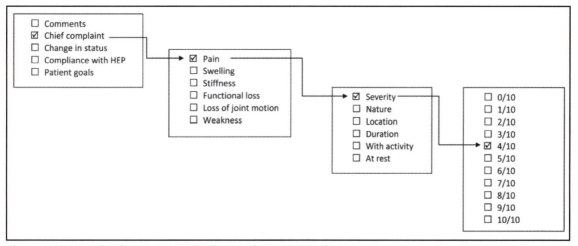

Figure 3-7. Sample electronic medical record (EMR) interface.

- TherAssist (www.therassist.com)
- Therapy Source (http://sourcemed.net)
- QuickNotes (www.qnotes.com)

The APTA and Cedaron Medical Incorporated joined forces to create APTA Connect, a computerized documentation package that can manage scheduling, documentation, and patient demographics. It can link to a national outcomes database, help communicate with other providers, provide patient management reports, and link to the current billing system.[20] For more information on APTA Connect or Cedaron Medical Incorporated you can visit the following Web sites:

- APTA (www.apta.org/CONNECT)
- Cedaron Medical Inc: (www.cedaron.com/apta-connect-features)

Areas of concern with computer-based documentation are security and patient confidentiality, especially when documentation software resides on a server or when health information will be transmitted electronically. The Health Insurance Portability and Accountability Act (HIPAA)[21] provides federally regulated standards for handling individually identifiable health information during electronic transmission. This legislation requires that facilities adopt privacy policies and procedures for maintaining secure patient records so they are not accessible to unauthorized personnel.[22] HIPAA will be discussed in more detail in Chapter 11.

IDEA, IFSPs, AND IEPs

The Individuals with Disabilities in Education Act (IDEA)[23] is a federal law that governs states to provide a free appropriate public education for all children with disabilities residing in the state between birth to age 21. From birth to age 3, the child is covered under IDEA Part

C. Children who are considered "at risk" for developmental delay are referred to the program, and an initial evaluation is completed to determine a child's eligibility.[24] If the child is eligible for services under this legislation, he or she receives an Individualized Family Service Plan (IFSP). This is a special kind of multidisciplinary documentation that is reviewed on an annual basis to address the needs of the child. It includes the child's present level of development, family concerns, results of outcome measures, anticipated goals, and kinds of services to be provided.[24] A model IFSP can be found at http://idea.ed.gov/part-c/search/new.

Once the child turns 3, he or she may be eligible for coverage under IDEA Part B.[24] This coverage lasts until age 21 as long as certain eligibility requirements are met. Children and adolescents receive services under Part B to meet their educational needs and allow them to function in a general education environment. Under Part B of IDEA, there is also a specialized kind of documentation known as an IEP, or an Individualized Education Plan. Like the IFSP, the IEP includes the child's current academic and functional levels, a statement of his or her measurable goals, and services that will be provided. The IEP also includes special accommodations necessary for the child to improve chances for success.[24] The IEP is also reviewed on an annual basis, at minimum. The web link http://idea.ed.gov/explore/home provides resources including training for individuals involved in programs for school-aged children. Physical therapy services provided to children in the school system are geared toward enhancing the child's function in the school in order to meet his or her educational needs. Services provided under this model are unique and differ from the medical model where physical therapy services are most often delivered. Examples of school-based services include meeting seating and positioning needs and addressing mobility issues in and around the school. A child who is getting services in the school system under an IEP may also be receiving outpatient physical therapy to address his or her medical needs.

Both the IFSP and IEP are somewhat analogous to the PT's initial plan of care in the medical model in that they serve as an outline of the expected outcomes and delineate services to be provided. Daily documentation in these settings also occurs at each encounter. In these settings, the documentation format often used is the Problem-oriented format. Using this format, the PT or PTA can describe the treatment provided that is aimed at meeting the annual goal.

REFERENCES

1. Quinn L, Gordon J. *Functional Outcomes: Documentation for Rehabilitation*. St. Louis, MO: Saunders; 2003.
2. Weed LL. *Medical Records, Medical Education, and Patient Care: The Problem-Oriented Medical Record as a Basic Tool*. Chicago, IL: Year Book Medical Publishers; 1970.
3. Reinstein L. Problem-oriented medical record: experience in 238 rehabilitation institutions. *Arch Phys Med Rehabil*. 1977;58:398–401.
4. Reinstein L, Staas WE, Marquette CH. A rehabilitation evaluation system which complements the problem-oriented medical record. *Arch Phys Med Rehabil*. 1975;56:396–399.
5. Milhous RL. The problem-oriented medical record in rehabilitation management and training. *Arch Phys Med Rehabil*. 1972;53:182–185.
6. Mcintyre N. The problem-oriented medical record. *Br Med J*. 1973;2:598–600.
7. Feinstein AR. The problems of the "problem-oriented medical record." *Ann Intern Med*. 1973;78:751–762.
8. Dinsdale SM, Mossman PL, Gullickson G, Anderson TP. The problem-oriented medical record in rehabilitation. *Arch Phys Med Rehabil*. 1970;51:488–492.
9. White JA. Managing care. Documentation: making it meaningful. *Physical Therapy Case Reports*. 2000;3(2):78–79.
10. Clifton DW. "Tolerated treatment well" may no longer be tolerated. *PT Magazine*. 1995;3(10):24.
11. Abeln SH. Improving functional reporting (utilization review). *PT Magazine*. 1996;4(3):26, 28–30.
12. Blecker D. Building better patient notes by using templates. *ACD-ASIM Ob*. 1998;18(9):32.
13. Feige M. Establishing standard rehabilitation evaluation forms. Arizona Association for Home Care. *Caring*. 1992;11(8):40–44.
14. American Physical Therapy Association. *The Guide to Physical Therapist Practice*. Alexandria, Va: American Physical Therapy Association; 2001. Available at: guidetoptpractice.apta.org. Accessed February 18, 2012.
15. American Physical Therapy Association. Defensible documentation for patient/client management. Available at: http://www.apta.org/Documentation/DefensibleDocumentation. Accessed February 1, 2012.
16. Lewis DK. Do the write thing: document everything. *PT Magazine*. 2002;10(7):30–34.
17. Abeln SH. Liability awareness. Reporting risk check-up. *PT Magazine*. 1997;5(10):38–42.
18. U.S. National Library of Medicine. 2011AA Minimum Data Set, 3.0 source information. Available at: http://www.nlm.nih.gov/research/umls/sourcereleasedocs/current/LNC_MDS30/. Published May 19, 2011. Updated November 15, 2011. Accessed January 28, 2012.
19. Brimer M. Focus on technology: making the move to electronic documentation. *PT Magazine*. 1998;6(10):58–62.
20. American Physical Therapy Association. APTA connect. Available at: http://www.apta.org/CONNECT/. Accessed April 20, 2011.
21. U.S. Department of Health and Human Services. Health information privacy. Available at: http://www.hhs.gov/ocr/privacy/. Accessed January 28, 2012.
22. Ravitz KS. The HIPAA privacy final modified rule. *PT Magazine*. 2002;10(11):21-25.
23. Individuals with Disabilities in Education Act of 2004, PL 108-446. 108th Congress (2004). Available at: http://idea.ed.gov/download/statute.html. Accessed February 2, 2012.
24. U.S. Department of Education. Building the legacy: IDEA 2004. Available at: http://idea.ed.gov/. Accessed February 2, 2012.

REVIEW QUESTIONS

1. List 4 types of documentation formats used in physical therapy.

2. Describe similarities and differences between narrative notes, POMRs, SOAP notes, and FORs.

3. Describe advantages and disadvantages of narrative notes, POMRs, SOAP notes, and FORs.

4. What type of information is found in the S, O, A, and P portions of a SOAP note?

5. When using SOAP and POMR formats, where should you place information provided by the patient's family?

6. What are positive and negative aspects of using forms and templates?

7. What are the positive and negative aspects of using an EMR?

8. What is HIPAA? Why is it important with regards to the EMR?

9. Do you think that general computer anxiety would hinder use of computerized documentation? Why or why not?

10. What could clinics provide to their staffs to help reduce computer anxiety when implementing computerized documentation or when training new staff?

APPLICATION EXERCISES

I.   Answer the following questions.

1.   Research some of the computerized documentation packages listed in this chapter. What are the some of the associated benefits of using these as indicated by the company? What is the cost? What is the policy on technical support and upgrades? Do they appear to be user-friendly? Why or why not?

2.   Research APTA Connect. What does it offer? What are some of the advantages and disadvantages of having standardized computer software across a variety of clinics?

3.   Talk to clinicians in your area about documentation formats used at their facilities. What do they like or dislike about documentation formats currently used? What other formats have they tried? What would be the ideal documentation format?

4.   Your supervising PT has asked you to work with a patient with the following problems: flaccid left upper extremity, weakness in left lower extremity, dependence with ambulation, requires assist for all transfers, unable to perform self-care or home management skills.

(a)   List 3 questions that you could ask this patient when initiating a treatment session to elicit information for the subjective portion of a SOAP note.

(b)   What are 3 tests, measurements, or functional activities you should document on this patient?

(c)   Compare and contrast SOAP, POMR, and FOR for this patient. What would be the same in all 3? What would be different? Which of these documentation formats would be most difficult to complete for this patient?

II.   Read each statements and determine whether it would belong in the S, O, A, or P portion of a SOAP note.

1.____ Gait: Ambulated 50' x 2 WBAT (R) LE with min (A) x 1 and verbal cues to advance the (R) LE.

2.____ Pt. reports that the HEP has helped improve ROM.

3.____ Pt. will RTC 2x/wk for the next 4 wks.

4.____ Transfers: bed to and from chair with mod (A) x 2.

5.____ Pt. progressing toward goals set on the initial evaluation.

6.____ Pt.'s wife stated that she has been assisting the pt. with his HEP.

7.____ Speak with the PT about possible re-eval. 2° to pt.'s rapid progress.

8.____ AROM: (R) knee 0–135°.

9.____ Improvements in knee ROM allow pt. to sit without difficulty and ascend and descend stairs with less difficulty.

10.____Pt. feels that he is benefiting from the strengthening exercises in that he is now able to open jars and lids (I).

11.____Pt. will be seen for bid gait training.

12.____Pt. c/o inability to move her (L) UE and LE.

13.____Pt. denies use of assistive prior to admission.

14.____Gait distance improved from 25' to 150' over the last week.

15.____Pt. demonstrating (L) neglect making her unsafe during gait and transfers.

16.____Muscle Performance: All (R) LE strength is 5/5.

17.____Vitals: HR 95 bpm, RR 12, and BP 140/95.

18.____Pt. has improved ability to transfer in/out of bed since initial visit.

19.____Will contact PT about possible d/c evaluation as pt. is no longer benefiting from the intervention.

20.____Pt.'s endurance is poor 2° to COPD.

21.____C/O inability to brush teeth and eat with the (R) hand 2° to decreased AROM of the (R) elbow.

22.____Pt. is unable to drive or perform safe community mobility at this time.

23.____Edema in the (R) ankle has decreased 2 cm.

24.____Pt. dons/doffs prosthesis (I)

25.____Wound appearance: 100% red, healthy granulation tissue with minimal drainage.

III. Of the above statements, which would be considered functional and appropriate using FOR?

IV. Of the above statements, which link intervention, impairment, and function?

Chapter 4

The Physical Therapy Process

Rebecca McKnight, PT, MS

CHAPTER OBJECTIVES

After reading this chapter, the student will be able to do the following:

1. Describe the physical therapy process.
2. Discuss the various ways patients enter the physical therapy care system.
3. List the 5 elements of the patient/client management model.
4. Define and describe each of the 5 elements of the patient/client management model.
5. Discuss the roles of the physical therapist (PT) and physical therapist assistant (PTA) within the patient/client management mode.
6. Describe the PTA's responsibilities related to patient care, documentation, and communication.

INTRODUCTION

Sadie had come to terms with the fact that she has multiple sclerosis (MS). After all, she had seen her aunt Linda, who also was diagnosed with MS, living a fruitful and productive life even if she had to make some changes in her daily routine. This did not, however, keep Sadie from getting frustrated with some of the new issues she had to face. Most recently she had been having difficulties with fatigue, which had been hindering her ability to function at work. More frustrating than fatigue, however, were the new symptoms of clumsiness affecting her arms and legs and causing her difficulty with most of her activities. Upon her neurologist's suggestion, Sadie had been admitted to the local hospital for treatment. After returning home from the hospital, Sadie was still experiencing difficulties with her daily tasks. Her neurologist
recommended that Sadie seek physical therapy services to address her coordination and balance issues. Sadie sat in front of her computer with a list of area physical therapy clinics and began to research each to see whether any of the PTs had experience with working with individuals with her problems.

To actively participate in the provision of physical therapy services efficiently and with confidence, you must start with an understanding of the entire physical therapy care process. This will enable you to appreciate the role you will play in the provision of physical therapy services and the role of your supervising PT(s). Based upon this, you will begin to grasp how integral communication is to the entire physical therapy care process and how essential effective documentation is in ensuring patients "receive appropriate, comprehensive, efficient, and effective quality care"[1] (Figure 4-1).

THE PHYSICAL THERAPY PROCESS

The Guide to Physical Therapist Practice[1] outlines the physical therapy process through the physical therapist patient/client management model. This model describes the 5 elements necessary to ensure optimal outcomes of physical therapy services once an individual has entered into the physical therapy system. These essential components include examination, evaluation, diagnosis, prognosis, and intervention[1] (Table 4-1).

Patient Point of Entry

Individuals enter the physical therapy system by self-referral or through a referral by another health care

Erickson M, McKnight R. *Documentation Basics: A Guide for the Physical Therapist Assistant, Second Edition* (pp. 33-40)

Figure 4-1. The role of documentation in the physical therapy process.

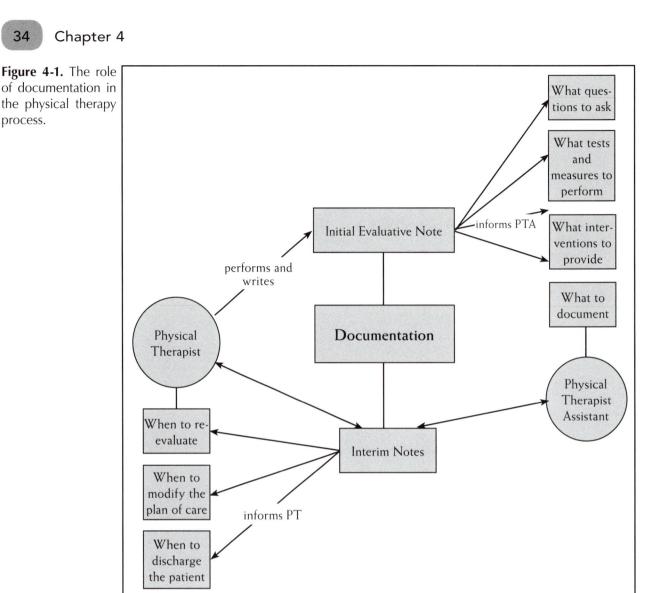

practitioner. Self-referral, also known as *direct access*, can only occur if the state practice act allows for it. As of March 2011, 46 states and the District of Columbia physical therapy practice acts allow for some degree of direct access.[2] Individuals in these states can legally seek physical therapy services, in at least some instances when they feel they have a need for physical therapy, without first obtaining a physician's referral. Frequently, patients enter the physical therapy system upon referral by another health care provider. Common referral sources include physicians, chiropractors, nurse practitioners, midwives, and dentists. A patient's initial introduction to physical therapy is often after hospitalization for disease or injury. At other times individuals will enter into the physical therapy care system through outpatient services, home health services, or school-based services.

The Patient/Client Management Model

Once an individual has entered the physical therapy system, the PT will initiate care through the examination/ evaluation process. This process is composed of 7 components: (1) history taking, (2) systems review, (3) tests and measures, (4) evaluation, (5) diagnosis, (6) prognosis, and (7) plan of care. During the history-taking portion of the examination, the PT gathers various pieces of information from the patient and from the patient's medical record, if one is available. This information allows the therapist to contextualize the patient's reason for seeking physical therapy services and ensures that the therapist attends to relevant factors that can affect the patient's prognosis. Types of data gathered during this process include the following[1]:

- General demographics (age, sex, race, etc)
- Social history
- Employment/work (job/school/play)
- Growth and development
- Living environment
- General health status
- Social/health habits (past and current)
- Family history
- Current condition(s)/chief complaint(s)

Table 4-1

THE FIVE ELEMENTS OF PATIENT/CLIENT MANAGEMENT

Element	Who/When	Includes	Source of Information	Purpose
1. Examination	Performed by the PT on all patients prior to the intervention	a.) History	Chart review Patient interview	Aids the PT in determining the most appropriate plan of care
		b.) Systems review	Examination of various body systems including: cardiovascular system, integumentary system, musculoskeletal system, neuromuscular system, communication, cognition, language, etc	
		c.) Tests and measurements	Range of motion measurements, gross muscle testing, sensation testing, girth, etc	
2. Evaluation	After the examination, the PT makes a clinical judgment based on findings			Allows others (including the PTA) insight to the anticipated level of improvement, intervention plan, and frequency and duration of services
3. Diagnosis	PT assigns a physical therapy diagnosis			
4. Prognosis (includes the Plan of Care)	PT determines the predicted level of improvement, treatment goals, expected outcomes, duration and frequency of treatment, and interventions to be used			
5. Intervention	Done by the PT or PTA to produce changes in the patient's condition	a.) Coordination, communication, and documentation	Working with other disciplines including physicians, occupational therapists, nurses, etc	Establish and maintain an open line of communication between disciplines
		b.) Patient/client-related instructions	Includes communicating with the patient and family	Informing patients and families
		c.) Procedural interventions	Includes things like hot packs, cold packs, range of motion exercises, strengthening exercise, gait training, transfer training, etc	Decrease inflammation, decrease pain, increase motion, etc

- Functional status and activity level
- Medications
- Other clinical tests (lab tests, radiology reports)

After obtaining a picture of the patient's condition and concerns, the PT will perform a systems review. During a systems review, the PT assesses the patient's overall medical health by reviewing the patient's cardiovascular/pulmonary system, integumentary system, musculoskeletal system, neuromuscular system, communication ability, affect, cognition, language, and learning style.[3] Based on information gathered during this process, the PT will select and perform appropriate tests and measures.[1] Test and measures are methods and techniques the therapist uses to gather data needed to determine the diagnosis and the intervention strategy. Tests and measures are also used later in patient/client management to evaluate outcomes and to note the patient's progress. The PT evaluates the information gathered during the examination process and makes clinical judgments about the findings to determine a physical therapy diagnosis and prognosis and to establish the plan of care. This clinical decision-making process is known as the *evaluation*.

The physical therapy plan of care is developed in collaboration with the patient and is based on the examination, evaluation, diagnosis, and prognosis. As indicated in the APTA "Defensible Documentation" materials, the plan of care includes the following[3]:

- Overall goals stated in functional, measurable terms that indicate the predicted level of improvement in function.
- A statement of interventions/treatments to be provided during the episode of care.
- Duration and frequency of service required to reach the goals.
- Anticipated discharge plans (may be part of the prognosis or written separately).

As indicated, every physical therapy plan of care must include succinct, "measurable and time limited"[1] goals written in functional terms. Goals serve as the tool to which outcomes are compared. This allows for assessment of the effectiveness of the plan of care and determination of the patient's progress. A well-written plan of care also delineates the interventions, treatment parameters, purpose of the interventions, progression parameters, and, if indicated, precautions.

Once the plan of care has been established, direct intervention can begin. A properly constructed physical therapy plan of care will incorporate appropriate interventions to ensure optimal outcomes and should include the following 3 components: (1) coordination, communication, and documentation; (2) patient-related instruction; and (3) procedural interventions.[1] Historically, when discussing a physical therapy plan of care, the emphasis has been placed on the physical agents or therapeutic activities planned. This correlates with the third component (procedural interventions) of a properly constructed physical therapy plan of care. More recently, there has been a growing appreciation for, and a shift toward recognizing the importance of, the other 2 components (coordination, communication, and documentation and patient/client-related instructions) of the physical therapy process. The patient/client management model clearly points to their inclusion into the plan of care.

As physical therapy interventions are initiated, the patient's progress toward the established goals (outcomes) is monitored. At various times within the process, re-examination may occur to formally document the patient's status and progress, or lack thereof. Based upon the findings from the re-examination, the PT may alter the plan of care. As part of the plan of care, the PT will develop discharge plans. Depending upon a variety of variables (the environment, the established goals, the patient's progress, and the prognosis), the plan may include transfer to another therapy service in another environment (acute rehab, skilled nursing, outpatient, or home health). When established goals are met, discharge from an episode of care occurs. Additionally, discontinuation of physical therapy services may occur without established goals being achieved. When this happens, the PT should document why the established goals were not met.[3] Upon discharge or discontinuation, the patient/client may be given a home exercise program or may be placed on a maintenance therapy program to maintain maximum functional capabilities in the absence of skilled therapeutic intervention. The establishment of a home exercise program, whether during the episode of physical therapy care or at the conclusion of physical therapy services, should be a part of the plan of care established by the PT.

PHYSICAL THERAPIST AND PHYSICAL THERAPIST ASSISTANT ROLES

APTA's *Direction and Supervision of the Physical Therapist Assistant*[4] clearly outlines the roles that the PT and PTA play within the patient/client management model. The PT is the recognized professional who establishes, guides, and directs all aspects of the provision of physical therapy services. It is the responsibility of the PT to interpret referrals; perform the initial examination and evaluation; establish the physical therapy diagnosis, prognosis, and plan of care (including goals and a discharge plan); and determine which interventions require the clinical decision-making skill of a PT and which interventions can be provided by a PTA. In addition, the PT is responsible for re-examination of the patient and revision of the plan of care when indicated. The PT is also directly responsible for ensuring appropriate documentation for all physical therapy services.[10]

As a PTA, your role in patient care activities will be within the intervention portion of the patient/client management model. You will implement selected interventions of the plan of care as directed by the PT. You will play an integral role with all 3 aspects of the intervention and should be prepared to participate in coordination, communication, and documentation; patient-related instruction; and procedural interventions. You must be able to utilize sound clinical judgment regarding the patient's readiness to engage in the selected interventions and the patient's response(s) to the intervention(s) being providing. You will need to determine when to consult with the PT about the patient's status and progress or lack thereof. Throughout the provision of interventions you will also need to perform appropriate tests in order to collect data to determine the patient's appropriateness to engage in selected interventions and to provide information useful in determining the patient's progress toward the goals established by the PT. As a PTA, you will be able to modify details of the treatment program, as directed by the supervising PT, to ensure the greatest efficiency and effectiveness in progressing the patient within the established plan of care or to ensure the patient's safety and comfort while engaged in the interventions being provided (Figure 4-2).[4]

Whether interventions are provided by the PT directly or by a PTA, the PT remains responsible for all aspects of the physical therapy service. As a PTA, you will be responsible for only providing the patient care interventions that are directed to you by the patient's PT. You will share the responsibility with the PT for guaranteeing that you only provide patient care interventions within your education and skill level and within legal parameters for the state in which you practice.[5-7] It will also be your responsibility to clearly and accurately document all patient care activities that you provide.[7,10]

For the provision of physical therapy services to be efficient and effective, a positive working relationship must exist between the PT and the PTA. This type of relationship is characterized by trust and mutual respect, as well as an appreciation for individual differences. A hallmark of a good working relationship is excellent communication.[8,9]

COORDINATION, COMMUNICATION, AND DOCUMENTATION

To ensure optimal outcomes from physical therapy services, it is imperative that appropriate coordination of services and communication related to those services occurs. Both of these components can be facilitated through, and should (at a minimum) be outlined in, concise documentation. Collaboration of services includes working with a variety of health care providers and, most important, the patient and the patient's family/support structure. Collaboration only occurs in the presence of rich communication. To be able to function within the health care delivery system you will need to effectively communicate with other members of the health care delivery team. Effective communication includes appropriate verbal and nonverbal communication as well as accurate documentation. Accurate and effective documentation will provide the foundation upon which all clinical activity occurs.

REFERENCES

1. American Physical Therapy Association. *The Guide to Physical Therapist Practice.* Alexandria, Va: American Physical Therapy Association; 2001. Available at guidetoptpractice.apta.org. Accessed February 18, 2012.
2. American Physical Therapy Association. FAQs: direct access at the state level. Available at: http://www.apta.org/StateIssues/DirectAccess/FAQs/. Accessed May 24, 2011.
3. American Physical Therapy Association. Defensible documentation: components of documentation within the patient/client management model. Available at: http://www.apta.org/Documentation/DefensibleDocumentation/. Accessed May 24, 2011.
4. American Physical Therapy Association. *Direction and Supervision of the Physical Therapist Assistant.* HOD P06-05-18-26. Available at: http://www.apta.org/uploadedFiles/APTAorg/About_Us/Policies/HOD/Practice/Direction.pdf. Accessed May 24, 2011.
5. American Physical Therapy Association. *A Normative Model of Physical Therapist Assistant Education.* Alexandria, Va: American Physical Therapy Association; 2007.
6. American Physical Therapy Association. *Minimum Required Skills of Physical Therapist Assistant Graduates at Entry-Level.* BOD G11-08-09-18. Available at: http://www.apta.org/uploadedFiles/APTAorg/About_Us/Policies/BOD/Education/./MinReqSkillsPTAGrad.pdf. Accessed May 24, 2011.
7. American Physical Therapy Association. Standards of ethical conduct for the physical therapist assistant. Available at: http://www.apta.org/uploadedFiles/APTAorg/About_Us/Policies/HOD/Ethics/Standards.pdf. Accessed May 24, 2011.
8. Holcomb S. Recipe for effective teamwork: why some PT/PTA pairings thrive, to patient's ultimate benefit. *PT Magazine.* February 2009. Available at: http://www.apta.org/PTinMotion/2009/2/PTAViewpoint/. Accessed February 18, 2012.
9. American Physical Therapy Association. PT/PTA teamwork: models in delivering patient care. Available at: http://www.apta.org/SupervisionTeamwork/Models/. Accessed May 24, 2011.
10. American Physical Therapy Association. *Guidelines: Physical Therapy Documentation of Patient/Client Management.* BOD G03-05-16-41. Available at: http://www.apta.org/uploadedFiles/APTAorg/About_Us/Policies/BOD/Practice/DocumentationPatientClientMgmt.pdf. Accessed May 24, 2011.

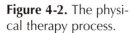

Figure 4-2. The physical therapy process.

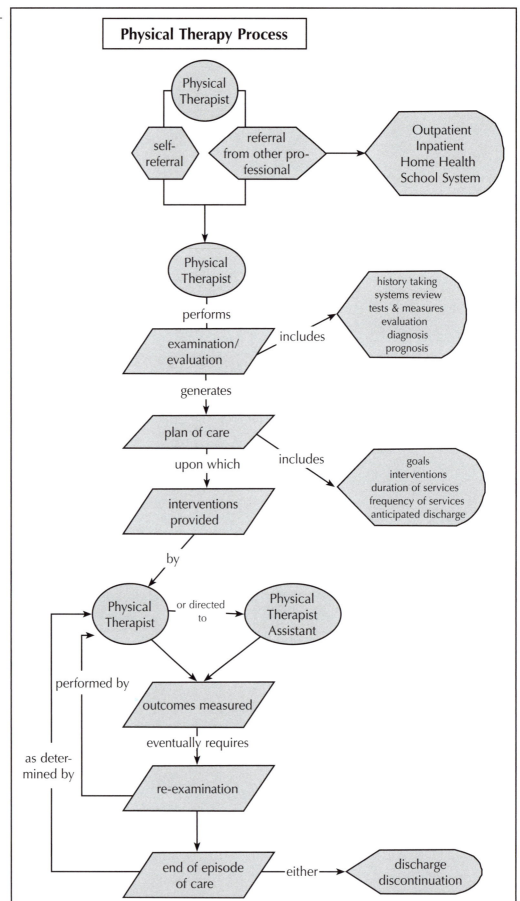

REVIEW QUESTIONS

1. Create a concept map (different from the one in the text) that outlines the physical therapy process.

2. Discuss various ways in which patients enter into the physical therapy care system.

3. Define and describe the 5 elements of the patient/client management model.

4. Next to each component of the patient/client management model indicate whether the PT, the PTA, or both participate(s) in that process.

    _____ Examination

    _____ Evaluation

    _____ Diagnosis

    _____ Prognosis

    _____ Intervention

5. Describe the role the PTA plays within the physical therapy process. List the responsibilities of the PTA within that role.

APPLICATION EXERCISES

I. Reference the physical therapy practice act for your state of residence for language regarding direct access. Does your state allow for direct access? Are there any restrictions or provisions related to direct access in the practice act?

II. Reference the physical therapy practice act for your state or residence for language regarding documentation. What are the responsibilities of the physical therapist assistant regarding documentation? What, if any, are the restrictions placed upon the physical therapist assistant regarding documentation? Compare your state practice act with a practice act from a different state. What are the similarities? What are the differences? Discuss how these differing requirements can impact the operation of physical therapy in a variety of settings.

III. Interview a friend or family member who has received physical therapy services. Ask him or her to describe how he or she entered the physical therapy care system. Ask him or her to describe the process as he or she remembers it. Compare the information you receive with the experiences reported by other interviews performed by your classmates.

Chapter 5

Interpreting the Initial Evaluation

Rebecca McKnight, PT, MS

CHAPTER OBJECTIVES

After reading this chapter, the student will be able to do the following:

1. List types of information that can be found in each component of an initial evaluative note.

2. List questions the PTA should ask when reviewing the evaluative note to guide decision related to provision of selected interventions.

3. Locate and use information in the initial evaluative note to determine which interventions are to be provided and how those interventions need to be performed.

4. Locate and use information in the initial evaluative note that will assist the PTA in judging the patient's performance and outcomes and determining what course of action needs to be taken.

INTRODUCTION

It was a bright July morning. Sarah approached the outpatient physical therapy clinic with a feeling of excitement and an air of expectation. This would be her first day of patient care as a licensed physical therapist assistant. As excited as she was, Sarah was also nervous. She knew she had an important role to play in her new position, and now she no longer had a clinical instructor or her college teachers helping her make decisions. Questions swirled through her mind as she walked in the door. "Am I really ready for this?" "Will I remember what I learned?" Her apprehension doubled as she met with John, her supervising physical therapist. As John began to discuss with Sarah the patient care activities he was directing her to perform that day, her questions

continued to trouble her. "Will I know what to do with the patients I will be working with?" "Will the interventions I provide be effective?" "Will John have confidence in my abilities?" Sarah's anxiety followed her throughout the morning until she sat down to review the chart for her first patient, Mrs. S.S. As she read the information about Mrs. S.S., she realized she knew exactly what to do, and she was able to approach her first patient with confidence that morning.

Sarah was able to have confidence as she began her day of patient care because she had a clear understanding of the physical therapy process and her role in it. Based on this understanding, Sarah knew what was expected of her, and she knew what to expect from John, her supervising physical therapist. Sarah's knowledge allowed her to be able to use the communication tool of the patient record to determine how she would proceed with Mrs. S.S.'s care that day.

DOCUMENTATION CONTINUUM IN PHYSICAL THERAPY

The APTA *Guidelines for Physical Therapy Documentation*[1] advises that documentation of physical therapy services should occur as follows: (1) at the initiation of services (the initial evaluation), (2) to detail all interventions provided, (3) to describe the patient's status and progress, (4) for all re-examinations or re-evaluations, and (5) at the end of the episode of physical therapy care. Documentation regarding physical therapy services begins with the physical therapist's initial evaluative note. The initial evaluative note will provide a clear picture of the patient by including pertinent history, risk factors, and results of tests and measures. The evaluative note will document the physical therapist's pro-

Erickson M, McKnight R. *Documentation Basics:*
A Guide for the Physical Therapist Assistant, Second Edition (pp. 41-60)
© 2012 SLACK Incorporated

Table 5-1

WHERE THE ELEMENTS OF THE PATIENT/CLIENT MANAGEMENT MODEL CAN BE FOUND IN A SOAP NOTE

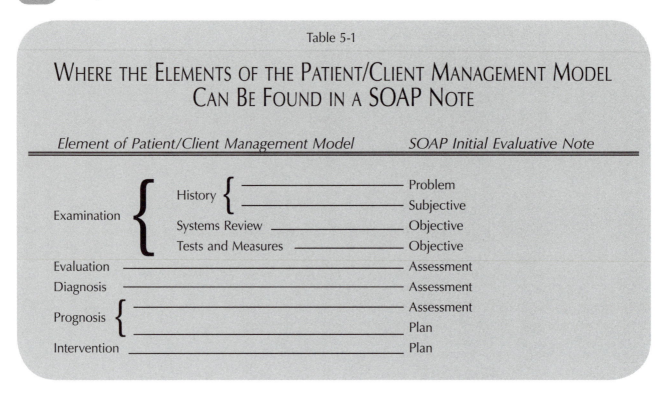

Element of Patient/Client Management Model	SOAP Initial Evaluative Note
Examination — History —	Problem
	Subjective
Systems Review	Objective
Tests and Measures	Objective
Evaluation	Assessment
Diagnosis	Assessment
Prognosis	Assessment
	Plan
Intervention	Plan

fessional judgment about the patient's condition, including the physical therapy diagnosis, prognosis, and anticipated goals. Finally, the evaluative note will include recommendations and a treatment plan.[1]

As a PTA, you will use the physical therapy initial evaluative note as a reference for each patient contact. The initial evaluative note should provide the framework upon which all patient-related activities you engage in are based. From the initial evaluative note, you should be able to obtain a clear picture of what is happening with the patient and how physical therapy services will be administered to address the patient's problems. You will have at least a general idea of what to anticipate when you work with the patient. This includes times when your interaction with the patient begins later in the patient's episode of care. Even though the patient might have had several physical therapy sessions, it will be important for you to review the initial evaluative note to gain a clear picture of the plan of care established by the physical therapist. In addition, you will need to review any subsequent documentation to gain an appreciation for how the patient has responded to the interventions and to see whether there have been any updates or revisions to the plan of care. Let's look at what a typical physical therapy evaluative note written in the SOAP format looks like and discuss how you can utilize this information to determine what you will do with the patient. Remember, even if an initial evaluative note is not documented in the SOAP note format, any patient record should have the same type of information. We will use the SOAP note format as a learning tool to help you distinguish what information you need

to attend to and how you will need to process the information to assist you in deciding how you should proceed with patient care activities.

SOAP INITIAL EVALUATIVE NOTE

You will find information related to the examination process in the problem, subjective, and objective sections of the evaluative note. Information about the evaluative process, as well as the diagnosis and prognosis, can be found in the assessment portion of the note. Finally, the plan for intervention will be documented primarily within the plan section (Table 5-1). We will look at each section individually, and then we will discuss how you will utilize the information to make decisions about what to do during your interactions with the patient.

Problem (Pr)

The problem section of a SOAP note is the first part of the initial evaluative note and provides information about the patient's reason for seeking physical therapy services. The problem can be derived from the history-taking portion of the examination, from the physician's referral, or from the medical record. The following information may be found in this section:

- Patient's chief complaint
- Medical diagnosis
- Physical therapy diagnosis
- Functional limitations

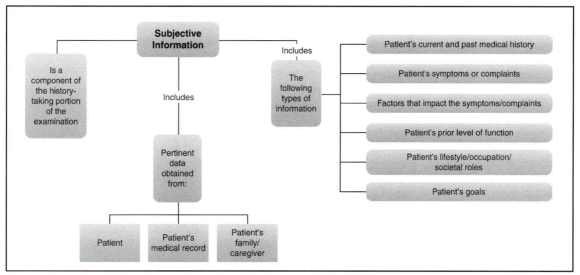

Figure 5-1. The Subjective section of a SOAP note. (Reprinted with permission from Erickson M, McKnight R, Utzman R. *Physical Therapy Documentation: From Examination to Outcome*. Thorofare, NJ: SLACK Incorporated; 2008.)

Example 5-1

Outpatient Physical Therapy Evaluation

Patient: S.S.
Age: 32 y.o.
Date of Eval: 7/14/11
Referral: PT to eval & tx
Referring Physician: Dr. Mark Long
Pr: ICD-9: 340—Multiple sclerosis—progressive remitting type
Pattern 5E: Impaired motor function and sensory integrity associated with progressive disorders of the central nervous system
Balance and coordination deficits

- Information gleaned from the medical record, such as:
  o Recent or past surgeries
  o Past conditions or diseases
  o Present conditions or diseases
  o Results of medical tests
- The physical therapy diagnosis can be listed as:
  o Preferred practice pattern
  o Impairments in body structures and functions
  o Limitations in activities and participation

In many settings, the problem section only includes the medical diagnosis and/or referral information with the remainder listed elsewhere (Example 5-1).[2]

Subjective (S)

The subjective section of a SOAP note provides all pertinent data that are obtained from the patient or the patient's family or caregiver. The subjective information is also a component of the history-taking portion of the examination (Figure 5-1). The following information can be found in this section:

- Patient's current and past medical history
- Patient's symptoms or complaints
- Factors that cause the symptoms or complaints
- Patient's prior level of function
- Patient's lifestyle/occupation/societal roles
- Patient's goals (Table 5-2)

As you begin to review physical therapy documentation in a variety of settings you will likely note that information gleaned from the patient's medical record can be recorded in a variety of areas. There is no standard regarding this practice. As noted above, some information might be found in the problem or subjective areas of the note. Additionally, some settings will have a separate section labeled "Medical History." On occasion the information is recorded in the objective section of the note. Regardless of where the information is documented, it is important for the physical therapist to indicate that the information was gleaned from a medical record instead of a patient's self-report (Example 5-2).

Objective (O)

The objective section of a SOAP note includes information related to tests performed or interventions provided (Figure 5-2). Objective data are a component of the examination. The physical therapist performs tests and gathers measurements and data through direct observation. Objective data are obtained through various methods and techniques such as range of motion measurements, gross muscle testing, sensation testing, girth measurements, and

Table 5-2

Subjective Types of Data

General Demographics
- Age
- Sex
- Race/ethnicity
- Primary language
- Education

Current Conditions/Chief Complaints
- Concerns that led the patient to seek the services of a physical therapist
- Current therapeutic interventions
- Mechanisms of injury or disease, including date of onset and course of events
- Onset and pattern of symptoms
- Patient/client, family, significant other, and caregiver expectations and goals
- Patient/client, family, significant other, and caregiver perceptions of patient's emotional response to the current situation
- Previous occurrence of the same complaints/symptoms
- Prior therapeutic interventions

Medical/Surgical History
- Cardiovascular
- Endocrine/metabolic
- Gastrointestinal
- Genitourinary
- Gynecological
- Integumentary
- Musculoskeletal
- Neuromuscular
- Obstetrical
- Prior hospitalizations, surgeries, and pre-existing medical and other health-related conditions
- Psychological
- Pulmonary

Medications
- For current condition
- Previously taken for current condition
- For other conditions

Other Clinical Tests
- Lab and diagnostic test
- Review of available records
  - Medical
  - Education
  - Surgical
- Review of other clinical findings
  - Nutrition
  - Hydration

Functional Status and Activity Level
- Current and prior functional status in self-care and home management
  - ADL
  - IADL
- Current and prior functional status:
  - Work (job/school/play)
  - Community
  - Leisure

Social History
- Cultural beliefs and behaviors
- Family and caregiver resources
- Social interactions, social activities, and support systems

Living Environment
- Devices and equipment
- Living environment and community characteristics
- Projected discharge destinations

General Health Status
- General health perception
- Physical function
  - Mobility
  - Sleep patterns
- Psychological function
  - Memory
  - Reasoning ability
  - Depression
  - Anxiety
- Role function
  - Community
  - Leisure
  - Social
  - Work
- Social function
  - Social activity
  - Social interaction
  - Social support

Social/Health Habits (Past and Current)
- Behavioral health risks
  - Smoking
  - Drug abuse
- Level of physical fitness

Growth and Development
- Developmental history
- Hand dominance

Family History
- Family health risks

Employment/Work
- Current and prior work
  - Job
  - School
  - Play
- Community
- Leisure

Example 5-2

S: *Demographics*: 32 y.o. right-handed Caucasian female; English speaking; completed 2 years of undergraduate college education

Social History: The pt. lives at home with her husband and 7 y.o. son. Three steps with a railing to enter her one level home. Pt.'s husband works during the day and her son goes to school. Her husband has been taking time off from work to stay with her during the day but will have to return to work this week. The pt. has various friends and family who have agreed to help her during the day until she is safe to be alone at home. Pt. normally active with taking son to after school activities.

Employment Status: She is normally employed as a bank teller but is unable to return to work at this time due to fatigue issues and "clumsiness."

General Health Status: Pt. reports prior to this last exacerbation she was in good health. Her primary activities included work, home care, and tending to her 7 y.o. son who participated in a variety of after school activities.

Medical History: Pt. reports she has not had any other issues that had required medical attention other than the birth of her son and typical illnesses (colds, flu, etc).

Current Condition: Pt. states she was diagnosed with progressive MS 2 years ago. On 7/1/11 she had an exacerbation of her MS that led her to be hospitalized for 3 days of IV anti-inflammatory medications. She was d/c'd to home on 7/4/11 with a wheeled walker. She was receiving PT while in the hospital. During her follow-up visit with her physician on 7/7/11 the pt. requested more PT due to balance and coordination problems. The pt. currently c/o "being unsteady on my feet," and being "clumsy with everything." Pt. reports she will be receiving OT to address coordination problems that interfere with daily functioning.

Functional Status: Pt. states she was previously (I) with all ADL and gait without an assistive device but has been utilizing a wheeled walker with assistance at home and a wheelchair for limited trips outside the home due to her unsteadiness. She reports having purchased the wheeled walker from a friend at church and borrowing the w/c from her mother-in-law.

Patient's Goals: The pt. states she would like to be able to walk without an assistive device, to return to work, and to be able to do housework.

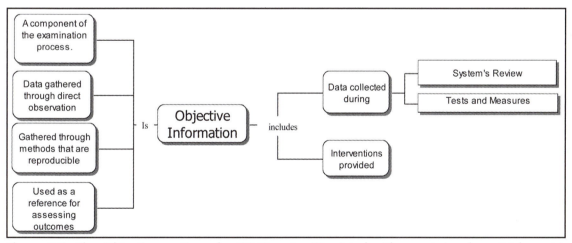

Figure 5-2. The Objective section of a SOAP note. (Reprinted with permission from Erickson M, McKnight R, Utzman R. *Physical Therapy Documentation: From Examination to Outcome*. Thorofare, NJ: SLACK Incorporated; 2008.)

functional tests. When possible, these methods are based on clearly defined procedures and are therefore reproducible. Using reproducible methods helps to ensure the validity and reliability of the data obtained. Objective data must have some measure of reliability and be useful in supporting the clinical decision-making process. The following types of information can be found in the objective section of the evaluative note (Table 5-3):

- Systems review
- Information gathered through:

Table 5-3

SUBHEADINGS FOR OBJECTIVE DATA

- Aerobic capacity
- Anthropometric characteristics
- Arousal, attention, and cognition
- Circulation
- Cranial and peripheral nerve integrity
- Environmental, home, and work barriers
- Ergonomics and body mechanics
- Gait
- Locomotion
- Balance
- Integumentary integrity
- Joint integrity or mobility
- Motor function
- Muscle performance

- Neuromotor development and sensory integration
- Orthotic, protective, and supportive devices
- Pain
- Posture
- Prosthetic devices
- Range of motion
- Reflexes
- Self-care and home management skills
- Sensation
- Ventilation/respiration
- Work, community, or leisure status and integration or reintegration (including IADL)[1]

Example 5-3

O: *Systems Review:*
    Cardiovascular/Pulmonary System: Unimpaired. BP: 120/78. HR: 78 bpm. RR: 16
    Integumentary System: Unimpaired
    Musculoskeletal System: Gross symmetry unimpaired. Gross ROM unimpaired. Gross strength impaired equally bilaterally UEs & LEs
    Neuromuscular System: Mobility impaired. Motor function impaired. Balance impaired
    Communication: Unimpaired
    Cognition: Unimpaired
Tests & Measures & Observation:
    Sensation: Pt. displays ↓ sharp/dull, proprioception & kinesthesia to (B) LEs from knees down.
    MMT: 4–/5 to 4+/5 throughout all four extremities utilizing standard test positions.
    Mobility: (I) with bed mobility, supine ↔ sit and sit ↔ stand requires SBA for safety due to ataxia. Pt. ambulates 200' with wheeled walker and min (A) on level surfaces, demonstrating truncal & (B) LE ataxia.
    Balance: Sitting static good–, dynamic fair+, standing static fair, dynamic fair–.
    Coordination: Pt. displays ataxia of all four extremities during functional tasks and during coordination tests including finger–nose–finger and heel–shin tests.
    Endurance: Fair for the above activities. Pt. fatigues after 15 minutes of activities.

- o Tests and measures
- o Observation
- Interventions provided
- Patient's response to interventions provided
- Education provided to the patient (Example 5-3)

Assessment (A)

The assessment section of a SOAP note provides the physical therapist's evaluation. In this section, the therapist assigns clinical meaning or value (evaluation) to the data collected during the examination process and documented within the subjective and objective sections of the SOAP note. The following will be found in the assessment section:

- Physical therapist's interpretation of S and O data (an overall summary of the patient)
- Goals
- Identification of impairments in body structures and functions
- Identification of limitations in activities and participation
- The relationship between body structure and functional impairments and limitations in activities and participation
- Physical therapy diagnosis or PT Practice Pattern (Table 5-4)
- Prognosis/rehabilitation potential
- Justification for goals/treatment plan

Table 5-4

PREFERRED PRACTICE PATTERNS

Musculoskeletal

Pattern A: Primary prevention/risk reduction for skeletal demineralization

Pattern B: Impaired posture

Pattern C: Impaired muscle performance

Pattern D: Impaired joint mobility, motor function, muscle performance, and range of motion associated with connective tissue dysfunction

Pattern E: Impaired joint mobility, motor function, muscle performance, and range of motion associated with localized inflammation

Pattern F: Impaired joint mobility, motor function, muscle performance, range of motion, and reflex integrity associated with spinal disorders

Pattern G: Impaired joint mobility, motor function, muscle performance, and range of motion associated with fracture

Pattern H: Impaired joint mobility, motor function, muscle performance, and range of motion associated with joint arthroplasty

Pattern I: Impaired joint mobility, motor function, muscle performance, and range of motion associated with bony or soft tissue surgery

Pattern J: Impaired joint mobility, motor function, muscle performance, and range of motion, gait, locomotion, and balance associated with amputation

Neuromuscular

Pattern A: Primary prevention/risk reduction for loss of balance and falling

Pattern B: Impaired neuromotor development

Pattern C: Impaired motor function and sensory integrity associated with nonprogressive disorders of the central nervous system—congenital origin or acquired in infancy or childhood

Pattern D: Impaired motor function and sensory integrity associated with nonprogressive disorders of the central nervous system—acquired in adolescence or adulthood

Pattern E: Impaired motor function and sensory integrity associated with progressive disorders of the central nervous system

Pattern F: Impaired peripheral nerve integrity and muscle performance associated with peripheral nerve injury

Pattern G: Impaired motor function and sensory integrity associated with acute or chronic polyneuropathies

Pattern H: Impaired motor function, peripheral nerve integrity, and sensory integrity associated with nonprogressive disorders of the spinal cord

Pattern I: Impaired arousal, range of motion, and motor control associated with coma, near coma, or vegetative state

Cardiovascular/Pulmonary

Pattern A: Primary prevention/risk reduction for cardiovascular/pulmonary disorders

Pattern B: Impaired aerobic capacity/endurance associated with deconditioning

Pattern C: Impaired ventilation, respiration/gas exchange, and aerobic capacity/endurance associated with airway clearance dysfunction

Pattern D: Impaired aerobic capacity/endurance associated with cardiovascular pump dysfunction or failure

Pattern E: Impaired ventilation and respiration/gas exchange associated with ventilatory pump dysfunction or failure

Pattern F: Impaired ventilation and respiration/gas exchange associated with respiratory failure

(continued)

Table 5-4 (continued)

PREFERRED PRACTICE PATTERNS

Pattern G: Impaired ventilation, respiration/gas exchange, and aerobic capacity/endurance associated with respiratory failure in the neonate

Pattern H: Impaired circulation and anthropometric dimensions associated with lymphatic system disorders

Integumentary

Pattern A: Primary prevention/risk reduction for integumentary disorders

Pattern B: Impaired integumentary integrity associated with superficial skin involvement

Pattern C: Impaired integumentary integrity associated with partial-thickness skin involvement and scar formation

Pattern D: Impaired integumentary integrity associated with full-thickness involvement and scar formation

Pattern E: Impaired integumentary integrity associated with skin involvement1 extending into fascia, muscle, or bone and scar formation

---

Example 5-4

A: Pt.'s motor deficits including balance, coordination, and strength deficits prevent her from mobilizing independently. The patient is unable to maintain her current employment and is not able to meet her roles as a wife and mother. The patient's rehab potential may be limited due to diagnosis of progressive remitting type MS. The patient's fatigue level will limit her participation but with continued efforts the patient may be able to achieve her stated goals. Will provide a 2-week trial of physical therapy intervention to determine the patient's potential.

STGs: To be achieved after 2 weeks of physical therapy.
1. (I) and safe with all transfer including sup ↔ sit & sit ↔ stand to allow patient greater (I) at home.
2. Pt. will ambulate with wheeled walker and SBA for safety on level surfaces and with CGA on uneven surfaces and stairs.
3. Increase general endurance so pt. can tolerate 30 minutes of functional and therapeutic activities to meet the above functional goals.
4. Increase strength ½ grade throughout all extremities to meet the above functional goals.
5. Improve coordination of extremities to meet the above functional goals.
6. Increase balance: static & dynamic sitting to good, static standing fair+ to meet the above functional goals.

LTGs: No LTGs set at this time until potential has been assessed over the next 2 weeks of therapy intervention.

- Explanation of any difficulties with obtaining S or O data
- Discussion of the patient's other problems (medical, social, financial) that can impact the patient's physical functioning or participation with a plan of care (comorbidities or complexities) (Example 5-4)

Plan (P)

The plan section of a SOAP note provides the written plan for physical therapy services and is part of the established plan of care. The following types of information may be found in the plan section:

- Plan for intervention activities to occur
  o Collaboration/communication
  o Patient-related education
  o Procedural interventions
- Frequency and duration of therapy services
- Treatment progression
- Suggestions for further testing, treatment, or referrals
- Plans for further assessment or reassessment
- Equipment needs
- Referral to other services (Example 5-5)

Example 5-5

P: Will be seen 3x/wk as an outpatient. Pt. will receive strengthening exercises, balance, & coordination activities, functional mobility training, and gait training. Will continue gait training with wheeled walker until (I) gait with wheeled walker is achieved then will progress to gait training with other (A) device as indicated.

HOW TO USE THE INITIAL EVALUATIVE NOTE

When you review the initial evaluative note you will want to glean specific information from each section to assist in determining what you need to do. To accomplish this, you need to start with a clear understanding of your role as a PTA. As described in Chapter 4, the PTA's role is in providing interventions as directed by the PT and as outlined in the established plan of care. You will want to focus on asking questions of the evaluative note that will facilitate your ability to carry out your role efficiently. As such, the first question you should ask is, "What interventions does the physical therapist want me to provide?" Answering this question first provides the appropriate context for you to process all other information found in the evaluative note, thus providing the foundation for all the decisions you will make related to the provision of the directed physical therapy interventions. You will also need to have a clear understanding of what the interventions are designed to address. Therefore, your next question should be, "What problem(s) is the intervention addressing?" For example, knowing that the PT wants you to help a patient with therapeutic exercises does not give you enough information to help you understand which therapeutic exercises you will need to provide or how they need to be provided. Are the therapeutic exercises to address a lack of muscle strength, a cardiovascular endurance issue, or a balance deficit? The answer to this question will significantly impact how you will proceed.

After this pair of questions has been answered, another pair of questions must be answered to bring further details to help you determine the approach you will take when providing the directed interventions. These questions are "What is the patient's current status regarding impairments in body structures or functions, functional capabilities and activity participation?" and "What are the goals that have been set by the physical therapist and patient regarding identified problems?" Following these questions you will want to ask, "What is the patient's diagnosis?" "What is the patient's prognosis?" "Are there any contraindications

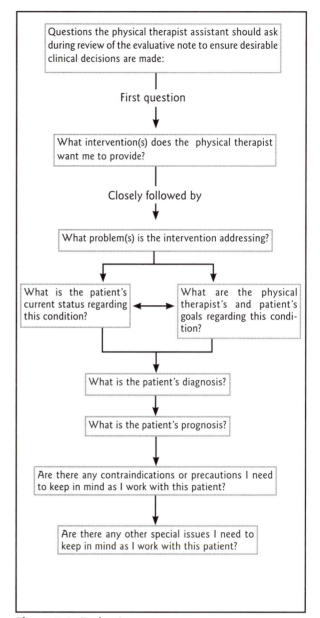

Figure 5-3. Evaluative note.

or precautions I need to keep in mind as I work with the patient?" and "Are there any other special issues I need to keep in mind as I work with this patient?" Special issues or considerations could include things like the patient's cognitive or psychological status. For example, it would be important to know whether the patient has a hearing or visual impairment in order to modify the therapy interventions to allow the patient to participate successfully in the therapy activities (Figure 5-3). The organization of questions in this figure does not imply that one question is more important than the other. Rather, this order helps to ensure that the PTA is processing the information found within the evaluative note in an efficient and effective manner to ensure that the best clinical decisions are made.

Table 5-5

INTERVENTIONS

Coordination, Communication, Documentation
Patient/Client-Related Instruction
Procedural Interventions
- Therapeutic exercise
- Functional training in self-care and home management, including activities of daily living (ADL) and instrumental activities of daily living (IADL)
- Functional training in work (job/school/play), community, and leisure integration or reintegration, including IADL, work hardening, and work conditioning
- Manual therapy techniques, including mobilization/manipulation
- Prescription, application, and, as appropriate, fabrication of devices and equipment (assistive, adaptive, orthotic, protective, supportive, or prosthetic)
- Airway clearance techniques
- Integumentary repair and protective techniques
- Electrotherapeutic modalities
- Physical agents and mechanical modalities[1]

Now that we have a clear picture of the questions that guide your review of the initial documentation, let's discuss where you will find this information within the note itself.

Question 1: "What intervention(s) does the physical therapist want me to provide?"

Although this question is often answered during a direct face-to-face conversation with the PT, it is important for you to review the evaluative note to discover what it says as well. On occasion, the PT might ask you to perform an intervention that is not included in the plan of care. In this case, it is your responsibility to clarify the need for the intervention with the PT and ask the PT to update the plan of care accordingly. On other occasions, you will need to determine which interventions to provide solely based upon the evaluative note. To find this information, you should start by looking the plan part of the note. In this section of the note, the physical therapist will have outlined the interventions to be provided (Table 5-5).

Question 2: "What problem(s) is the intervention addressing?"

As noted above, this question is imperative to help you determine in more detail how you will proceed when providing the intervention(s). Ideally, you will be able to find this information in the plan right alongside the interven-

tion. For example, the PT might write, "Patient to receive therapeutic exercise to address strength deficits in the right quadriceps." When this much detail is included in the plan, it is easier for you to determine how you will proceed. This level of detail helps you quickly determine which exercises you will likely instruct the patient to perform. Obviously there are more questions to answer, but you are well on your way to knowing how to proceed with this patient. On the other hand, the plan might not provide any information that helps delineate specifically what the interventions are for, or perhaps the patient has multiple areas of involvement that need to be addressed. For example, the therapist writes a broader intervention statement, such as, "Patient to receive therapeutic exercises to address muscle strength and endurance issues." In this case you will have more work cut out for you in your review to determine what muscles are in need of strengthening. You can also find information in the assessment section (within the problem list and the goals) to help determine what problem(s) the interventions are designed to address. If after review of the evaluative note you are still unclear of the purpose for the interventions, it is essential that you clarify this with the PT. Many interventions have the capacity of addressing more than one problem utilizing different parameters. For example, electrotherapeutic modalities can be utilized to address both pain and muscular weakness. A patient recovering from knee surgery could be dealing with both of these issues. If the therapist indicated use of electrotherapeutic modalities in the plan but did not specify for which problem, you would need to clarify this prior to utilizing the modality.

Questions 3 and 4: "What is the patient's current status regarding this condition?" and "What are the physical therapist's and patient's goal(s) regarding this condition?"

Information regarding the patient's current status should be reviewed in light of the established goals. This will help you get an understanding of exactly what you should expect from the patient and how you should be prepared to progress with the patient. This will also provide you with a clear expectation of how quickly the patient will be able to progress. Information regarding the patient's current status can be found in the objective portion of the note. Further insights regarding the patient's current status can be gleaned from the problem list and the narrative, or summary statement found in the assessment portion. Goals established by the PT are listed in the assessment section of the note with clearly detailed expected timelines for reaching the goals.

Questions 5 and 6: "What is the patient's diagnosis?" and "What is the patient's prognosis?"

When looking at the evaluative note to find the patient's diagnosis, you should remember to look for both the medical diagnosis (CVA, multiple sclerosis [MS], patella fracture, etc) as well as the physical therapy diagnosis. The physical therapy diagnosis can be a statement that relates impairment to function. The physical therapy diagnosis could also be indicated by a preferred practice pattern (see Table 5-4). The medical diagnosis may also be found in the problem section of the note. The physical therapy diagnosis will at times be found in the problem section as well, but it should always be found within the assessment component of the note.

The prognosis should be found as a direct statement within the assessment section of the note. The prognosis will be communicated by the goals and time frame in which the goals are to be met. This information will provide you with a general idea of what to expect from the patient. For example, in the patient case above, as soon as Sarah read that S.S. has a diagnosis of progressive remitting MS, she had a general idea of what to expect from the patient based on her knowledge of that disease process. Further information provided in the remainder of the note helped Sarah to fill in the details so she had a clearer picture of what to expect of S.S.'s status and performance.

> *Questions 7 and 8: "Are there any contraindications or precautions I need to keep in mind as I work with this patient?" and "Are there any other special issues I need to keep in mind as I work with this patient?"*

It is imperative for you to recognize and follow any contraindications and precautions. Often these will be directed by the physician, especially when related to recovery after a surgical procedure. When a contraindication is directed by the physician, it often is found within the problem component of the note. Additional precautions and contraindications might be found within the assessment or plan sections of the note. At times contraindications and precautions are not directly specified but rather it is expected that you will know standard contraindications or precautions associated with conditions commonly addressed with physical therapy services. For example, if a patient who is recovering from a CVA has diminished muscle performance in the musculature that surrounds the shoulder joint, it is expected that you will know appropriate precautions to take to limit subluxation and potential dislocation of the joint.

Therefore, when reading all components of the evaluative note you will want to ask yourself whether there is any information that would indicate specific contraindications or precautions you need to monitor during provision of the directed interventions.

There are numerous additional issues you might need to consider, and it is impossible to delineate all of them. A few examples follow to help demonstrate what types of things you will want to consider. First, upon review of the problem and subjective areas you might find information regarding comorbidities that can impact the patient's ability to participate in the interventions you have been directed to provide. For example, you might be asked to provide transfer training for a patient who has left-side weakness due to a recent stroke. The chart indicates that the patient has previously had a right transtibial amputation. This information will help you adjust your plan of action when making a decision related to how you will approach the transfer training activities. Second, psychological and emotional issues might also be recorded in the therapist's note, providing you with valuable insight that will help you adjust your approach. For example, elderly individuals who have sustained injuries due to a fall incident often deal with fear of falling issues that can significantly impact their ability to participate and progress in physical therapy. Because there is such a myriad of issues that can impact the provision of physical therapy, you will want to review the evaluative note for any potential issues so you can modify the intervention strategy or your approach to increase the likelihood for success.

ADDITIONAL QUESTIONS TO ANSWER

Once you have answered the above questions, you should have a good idea of how you will proceed with working with the patient. However, there are a few more questions you will want to ask prior to initiating the therapy session.

After you have a clear picture of what interventions you will provide and how you will provide them, you will want to ask what tests need to be performed prior to initiating the interventions. Data are gathered prior to beginning interventions for 2 basic reasons: first you will want to ensure that the patient's status indicates that it is safe to participate in the specific interventions you have been directed to provide. Second, you will want to gather any data that are essential to demonstrate the patient's response to the intervention being provided.

> *"What tests do I need to perform prior to initiating interventions to ensure the patient is safe and able to participate in the selected intervention(s)?"*

Two pieces of data that should be collected prior to initiating any therapy session are heart rate and blood pressure. These 2 pieces of data provide an important insight into the patient's physiologic status and safety for participating with physical therapy interventions. As you review the evaluative note, you need to identify whether the patient has a history of a cardiovascular condition or is taking any medications that can alter normal cardiovascular responses. This will help you be prepared to respond appropriately once you have gathered the patient's heart rate and blood pressure readings.

Other data might be important to gather to determine the patient's readiness to participate in the therapy session. This will be dependent upon the individual patient case. Examples include oxygenation saturation for individuals with a respiratory condition, pain ratings for individuals recovering from a musculoskeletal surgical procedure, and cognitive status for patients who have sustained a head injury due to trauma. Again, many other conditions exist that might require you to perform preintervention tests to determine the patient's ability to participate in the interventions. You will need to review the evaluative note to determine which tests you will need to perform, observations you need to make, or questions you need to ask of the patient.

"What additional tests do I need to perform to demonstrate the patient's response to the intervention(s) provided and the patient's progress toward the established goals?"

Other tests that you might need to perform prior to initiating the intervention include tests that will provide data regarding how the patient responds to the intervention being provided when pre- and postmeasurements are indicated. Just as it is important to measure heart rate and blood pressure to ensure it is safe for the patient to participate in physical therapy, baseline data are equally important in order to compare during and postintervention. No better data can be found to provide a picture of the patient's cardiovascular response to treatment. Pain ratings are also commonly utilized to determine the patient's response to the interventions during and after they are provided. Some interventions are directed toward pain management, and the patient's pain rating will need to be gathered pre- and postintervention to demonstrate the effectiveness of the intervention. At other times pain ratings are utilized to determine what the intensity of the intervention should be. The type of data needed depends upon the particular interventions being provided, the reason for the intervention, the goals, as well as the time frame in which goals are expected to be accomplished. You can speak to the PT if you are unsure how to gauge intervention intensity.

As you determine which tests you will need to perform, you will need to make a mental list of the equipment you will need (blood pressure cuff, stethoscope, etc). In addition, as you review the subjective information you will want to think about what questions you might want to ask the patient. In S.S.'s case, Sarah may want to ask how the assistance from friends and family has been working out.

Although the majority of tests that you will perform prior to providing interventions to gain "before" measurements will also be performed during and/or after the intervention to provide insight into the patient's response, you might also need to perform additional tests that are not performed prior to those interventions. Some of these data are not needed for each session, so it will be important to clarify with the PT whether a particular test needs to be performed during a given session. For example, to monitor S.S.'s progress toward the established goals and responses to the interventions provided, Sarah will observe S.S.'s functional mobility status and then will need to perform manual muscle testing (MMT) and balance and coordination testing at some point. During your review of the evaluative note, you will again want to add to your mental list any additional equipment you will need to gather to perform these tests and measures.

"What equipment will I need to be able to provide this intervention?"

Review of the objective and assessment portions of the note will help you determine what equipment you will need in order to provide the intervention. For example, upon review of S.S.'s evaluative note you know that in order to provide gait training activities you will want to ensure that there is a wheeled walker and gait belt available.

"What other information should I keep in mind?"

When reading the subjective portion of the note you also want to think about other pieces of information you want to be listening for as you provide your intervention. Frequently, patients share important information days or weeks after the initial evaluation. This information can be useful in providing a more efficient plan of care. For example, if S.S. were to share a history of a previous right arthroscopic knee surgery with occasional knee pain, Sarah would want to document this information in the patient's chart and communicate it to the supervising PT. This may help to explain discrepancies in strength gains between the legs if any are noticed in future sessions.

When you review the objective information, you want to picture in your mind how the patient will look and act. This will allow you to anticipate appropriate responses to therapeutic intervention and will help you identify inappropriate responses. As Sarah works with S.S., she will expect the patient to fatigue and will build rest breaks into the therapy session depending upon the level of activities performed. However, Sarah will not expect any specific complaints of pain. If S.S. begins complaining of localized pain in her left ankle, Sarah would know to consult with the PT.

As you read the assessment portion of the note, you will be able to outline in your mind how the patient should progress. This will guide you in the day-to-day decisions about what needs to happen with the patient. Review of the plan section will tell you the anticipated duration of the episode of care. Based upon John's assessment of S.S., Sarah would not be alarmed if the patient did not show significant improvements over the course of the treatment plan.

"Do I need to know anything else?"

The final question that you need to ask yourself is, "Is there any other information I need that is not found in the evaluative note?" If the answer is yes, you will want to seek out the information from the appropriate source (may or may not be the PT). For example, you know that the patient had lab work done earlier in the day. You will want to review the lab values to determine whether it is safe for the patient to participate in therapy or whether the PT needs to be contacted. It is imperative that you ask clarifying questions prior to initiating care to ensure the safety of the patient and to improve effectiveness of care. If the patient's initiating therapist is not available, you should ask the therapist providing supervision and direction for the patient on that particular day.

At this point it should be clear how important the evaluative note is in providing essential information to guide the PTA's decision-making process regarding interventions. You should also be able to appreciate the importance of providing timely and accurate interim notes regarding the therapy sessions you provide. Comprehensive documentation of care provided will help ensure effective and efficient physical therapy services are provided.

REFERENCES

1. American Physical Therapy Association. *Guidelines: Physical Therapy Documentation of Patient/Client Management.* BOD G03-05-16-41. Available at: http://www.apta.org/uploadedFiles/APTAorg/About_Us/Policies/BOD/Practice/DocumentationPatientClientMgmt.pdf. Accessed May 24, 2011.
2. American Physical Therapy Association. *The Guide to Physical Therapist Practice.* Alexandria, Va: American Physical Therapy Association; 2001. Available at guidetoptpractice.apta.org. Accessed February 18, 2012.

REVIEW QUESTIONS

1. For each of the following components of the patient/client management model, indicate where this information can be found within an initial evaluative note written in the SOAP note format. Write Pr for problem, S for subjective, O for objective, A for assessment, and P for plan.

    _____ Prognosis

    _____ Examination: History-taking

    _____ Evaluation

    _____ Intervention

    _____ Examination: Systems review

    _____ Diagnosis

    _____ Examination: Tests and measures

2. For each of the following types of information that may be found in a physical therapy evaluative note, indicate where the information would be documented in the SOAP note format. Write Pr for problem, S for subjective, O for objective, A for assessment, and P for plan.

    _____ Rehabilitation potential

    _____ Patient education provided

    _____ Medical diagnosis

    _____ Patient's complaints

    _____ Equipment needed

    _____ Goals

    _____ Recent surgeries

    _____ Patient's prior level of function

    _____ Interventions provided

    _____ Results of tests

3. Discuss the importance of documenting patient education and communication within the intervention provided in the patient/client management model.

4. List the questions the PTA should ask when reviewing the evaluative note to guide interventions.

5. Discuss the importance of starting the review of the evaluative note by determining what interventions the physical therapist wants you to provide.

APPLICATION EXERCISES

I.   Using the case examples in Examples 5-6 through 5-8, practice reviewing initial evaluative notes to prepare for a treatment session. Utilize the questions as outlined in this chapter.

1.   "What interventions does the physical therapist want me to provide?"

2.   "What problem(s) is the intervention addressing?"

3.   "What is the patient's current status regarding this condition?"

4.   "What are the physical therapist's and patient's goal(s) regarding this condition?"

5.   "What is the patient's diagnosis?"

6.   "What is the patient's prognosis?"

7.   "Are there any contraindications or precautions I need to keep in mind as I work with this patient?"

8.   "Are there any other special issues I need to keep in mind as I work with this patient?"

9.   "What tests do I need to perform prior to initiating interventions?"

10. "What additional tests do I need to perform to demonstrate the patient's response to the interventions provided and the patient's progress toward the established goals?"

11. "What equipment will I need to be able to provide this intervention?"

12. "What other information should I keep in mind?"

13. "Do I need to know anything else?"

Example 5-6

Anytown Community Hospital: Skilled Nursing Facility

Physical Therapy Evaluation
Patient: J.M.
Age: 76 y.o.
Date: 04/04/10
Referral: Physical therapy for gait and strengthening. Anterior hip precautions, WBAT
Referring Physician: Dr. Mark John
Pr: (L) THA 03/30/10. HTN; 2 previous TIAs approx. 1 year ago.
S: *Complaint:* The patient states he does have some soreness but in general his hip pain is less than before the surgery; rates pain as 1–2/10 and states it hurts worse at the end of the day.
      Living environment/Social Support: The patient reports he lives at home with his wife. His wife is generally in good health and is active in the community but pt. is concerned about being a "burden" on his wife when he returns home. Pt. states he has 3 steps with railing on one side to enter his one level home.
      Prior level of function/activities: The patient states he was previously (I) with ADLs and gait without (A) device; his hobbies include yard work and doing crossword puzzles; he is retired; pt. normally attended church twice a week and meet with friends for coffee 3–4 times a week; pt. enjoys fly fishing 3–4 times a month "depending upon the weather."
      Patient Goals: The patient states he would like to return to his previous level of activity and specifically is hoping to participate in a fishing tournament this fall.
O: *Systems Review:*
          Cardiovascular/Pulmonary System: Unimpaired. BP: 130/85. HR: 88 bpm. RR: 20
          Integumentary System: Healing scar (L) Hip, staples intact, no drainage noted
          Musculoskeletal System: Gross strength general decrease (B) UEs and (R) LE; (L) LE impaired due to recent surgery. Gross ROM (L) LE restricted due to orthopedic precautions; other extremities and trunk unimpaired
          Neuromuscular System: Balance & motor control unimpaired. Functional mobility impaired
          Communication: Unimpaired
          Cognition: Unimpaired   *(continued)*

Example 5-6 (continued)

Tests & Measures & Observation:

Strength: 4/5 to 4+/5 throughout (B) UEs and (R) LE. (L) hip musculature not tested at this time due to recent surgery. Appears 2/5 with functional mobility. (L) knee strength 3+/5, ankle strength 5/5.

Mobility: Scooting in bed min (A) to assist (L) LE. Supine ↔ sit with Mod (A) x 1, Sit ↔ stand with min (A) x 1.

Gait: Pt. ambulated 50' with walker and min (A) x 1 WBAT (L) LE. Pt. needed frequent v/c for proper walker placement 2° tendency to place walker too far in front of him.

Treatment: Initiated bed mobility training, transfer training, and gait training using front wheeled walker; AAROM to (L) LE, including ankle pumps, quad sets, ham sets, glut sets, SAQ, SLR, hip abd, and heel slides 2 x 10. Pt. required min (A) x 1 with SAQs and heel slides and mod (A) x 1 with SLRs and hip abd.

Pt. Education: Pt. was instructed in hip precautions. Pt. was able to repeat hip precautions after 10 minutes of alternate activities.

A: Pt's decreased strength (L) LE is limiting his functional (I). Pt. is unable to return home at this time due to dependence with mobility and need to learn hip precautions to protect recent THA surgery. This pt. is very motivated and does not have significant comorbidities and therefore has excellent rehab potential.

Problem List:

1. Decreased strength (L) LE
2. Dependent mobility
3. Dependent gait
4. Does not know hip precautions for functional tasks

STGs: To be met within 2 days

1. Pt. will require SBA-CGA with all bed mobility & transfers.
2. Pt. will ambulate 100' with walker & CGA on level surfaces.
3. Increase (L) LE strength to 3/5 throughout hip and 4−/5 knee to be able to meet the above functional goals.
4. Pt. will be able to verbalize all hip precautions and will demonstrate understanding of precautions during basic transfers and gait activities.

LTGs: To be met within 7 days to allow the patient to return home with his wife.

1. Pt. will be (I) with all bed mobility & transfers and car transfers with min (A) of wife.
2. Pt. will ambulate 200' with walker (I) on level surface & up and down 3 steps utilizing railing on one side with SBA of wife.
3. Increase (L) LE strength to 3+/5 throughout hip and 4/5 knee to be able to meet the above functional goals.
4. Pt. will display good understanding of hip precautions during all functional activities including car transfers and gait on stairs.

P: PT BID, for ROM/strengthening exercises, transfer training including car transfers, gait training including gait on stairs and education regarding hip precautions with all functional tasks.

Ted Orlando, DPT

Example 5-7

Anytown Community Hospital: Subacute Rehabilitation

Physical Therapy Evaluation

Patient: D.W.

Age: 68 y.o.

Date: 05/26/10

Referral: Physical therapy to evaluate and treat as advised

Referring Physician: Dr. Sue Morton

Pr: Brainstem CVA 05/21/10; Type 2 diabetes; (R) carotid endarterectomy 07/08, and three previous TIAs.

S: *Current Condition:* Pt. reports that on 05/21/10 she awoke to find she could not get herself out of bed. She had been experiencing feelings of fatigue and weakness the evening before and had gone to bed early. Pt.'s husband called emergency services and she was transported to the hospital where the diagnosis of brainstem CVA was made.

Patient Complaint: The pt. c/o weakness on the (R) side of her body and "clumsiness" with her (L) arm. She states she is unable to anything on her own at this point. The pt. admits to being very frustrated and just "wants to give up."

Living Environment/Social Support: Pt. reports she previously lived at home with her husband in a one-story ranch style home with 1 step to enter. The pt. and her husband have 3 children. One son lives in the area and can be available to assist some. The other 2 children do not live in the area. Her husband owns his own business as an electrician and will be able to cut back his "hours of work" to help her if needed.

Prior Level of Function/Activities: Pt. states she has always been a "housewife" and is sure her husband would be unable to "run the home." Pt's social activities include being involved in a reading club that meets monthly and going to church weekly. Pt. also reports she occasionally keeps her neighbor's children in the evenings. The children are 5 and 8 years old.

Patient's Goals: She states she and her husband are hoping that she can eventually return home. She would like to return to as many of her previous activities as possible but voices she understands she may need to use a cane, walker, or wheelchair to get around. Pt. is most concerned about being able to take care of her home including doing dishes, laundry, and general house cleaning tasks.

O: *Systems Review:*

Cardiovascular/Pulmonary System: BP: 128/70. HR: 74 bpm. RR: 20

Integumentary System: Unimpaired

Musculoskeletal System: Gross ROM unimpaired. Gross strength impaired throughout trunk and (B) UEs & LEs (R) > (L)

Neuromuscular System: Balance & motor control impaired throughout trunk and all 4 extremities. Functional mobility impaired for all tasks

Communication: Mild slurred speech. Pt. easily understood

Cognition: Unimpaired

Other: Urinary catheter noted

Tests & Measures & Observation:

Observation: Pt. grossly obese

Sensory: Pt. demonstrates normal light & gross touch, pain/thermal and diminished proprioception/kinesthesia on (L) and mildly diminished light & gross touch, pain/thermal, and proprioception/kinesthesia on (R) throughout trunk and extremities.

Tone: The patient displayed mild hypotonia (R) UE & LE and normal tone (L) UE & LE.

MMT:		(R)	(L)
Shoulder			
	Flexors	2/5	4/5
	Extensors	1/5	4/5
	Abductors	1/5	4/5
	Adductors	2/5	5/5
	Medial Rotators	2/5	5/5
	Lateral Rotators	1/5	4−/5

(continued)

Example 5-7 (continued)

		(R)	(L)
Elbow			
	Flexors	2/5	5/5
	Extensors	0/5	4+/5
Wrist			
	Flexors	1/5	4/5
	Extensors	0/5	4−/5
Grip		5#	28#
Hip			
	Flexors	1/5	4−/5
	Extensors	3/5	4−/5
	Abductors	0/5	4−/5
	Adductors	3+/5	5/5
Knee			
	Flexors	0/5	4/5
	Extensors	2+/5	5/5
Ankle			
	Dorsiflexors	0/5	4+/5
	Plantarflexors	1/5	5/5

Balance: Sitting static fair−, dynamic poor; Standing not assessed at this time.

Coordination: Unable to assess (R) side due to weakness. (L) UE & LE demonstrates diminished coordination with all activities. Note apraxia and pass pointing during exercises.

Bed Mobility: Max (A) x 1 with rolling and scooting in bed.

Transfers: Max (A) x 1 supine ↔ sit. Unable to perform sit ↔ stand at this time. Bed ↔ mat at this time is via Hoyer due to patient's large size, poor balance, and weakness.

A: This obese pt. has very severe functional disabilities. Pt. is motivated and pleasant to work with. Due to the severe deficits prognosis for significant recovery is poor; however, the pt. and her husband want to try to get the pt. back home. A trial of structured aggressive therapy is indicated to see how much functional return is possible for this pt. and to educate her husband on how to provide any necessary care.

Problem List:
1. Decreased strength (R) > (L)
2. Decreased coordination (L) UE & LE
3. Decreased balance
4. Dependent with all mobility

STGs: Within 2 weeks the pt. will display:
1. Mod (A) x 1 for bedmobility and supine ↔ sit.
2. Max (A) x 1 for bed ↔ w/c using slideboard transfer.
3. Fair static and fair− dynamic sitting balance.
4. Increase strength ½ grade throughout to be able to achieve functional goals.
5. Improve coordination (L) UE & LE to be able to achieve functional goals.

LTGs: Within 4 weeks the pt. will display:
1. Min (A) x 1 for bedmobility and supine ↔ sit.
2. Mod (A) x 1 for bed ↔ w/c using slideboard transfer.
3. Fair+ static and fair dynamic sitting balance.
4. Increase strength one grade throughout to be able to achieve functional goals.
5. Improve coordination (L) UE & LE to be able to achieve functional goals.

Pt.'s husband will:
6. Safely assist pt. with bed mobility and all transfers.

P: PT BID for neuromuscular re-education, strengthening exercises, endurance activities, mobility training, and family education. Will assess pt's equipment needs for home use and facility acquisition of the equipment. Pt. will require at minimum a wheelchair and a BSC. Prior to discharge recommend pt. & pt's husband stay in the independence apartment to assess their ability to manage in a "home like" environment. Anticipate continued therapy through home health services will be needed. If patient demonstrates good recovery over her rehab stay may recommend an extension of her stay to work toward greater independence.

Joe Jackson, DPT

Example 5-8

Anytown Community Hospital: Outpatient Rehabilitation Services

Physical Therapy Evaluation
Patient: B.H.
Age: 85 y.o.
Date: 09/26/10
Referral: PT for ROM and strengthening to the (L) elbow.
Referring Physician: Dr. Jeff Gordon
Pr: (L) Elbow fracture s/p ORIF 8/18/10; (L) hip fx s/p ORIF 1/08
S: *Current Condition:* Pt. states she broke her arm when she missed a step coming out of her house into her garage 08/18/10; pt.'s husband took her to the emergency room; she had surgery the same day and returned home the next day. During a follow-up visit to the doctor on 09/21/10 the cast was removed. Pt. states she is coming to PT to get her "arm working again."

Patient Complaint: Pt. reports her (L) UE seems to ache all the time especially over the weekend since her cast was removed. Pt. ranks her pain as 2/10 at rest, 3–4/10 with activities, 6–7/10 during stretching/ROM exercises. Pt. reports she still is occasionally using painkillers prescribed by the physician and reports relief of her pain with meds.

Living Environment/Social Support: Pt. lives at home with spouse. Denies any steps to negotiate. Pt. reports prior to accident she was (I) with ADLs and gait without (A) device. Pt. does own a walker from previous (L) LE surgery; pt. reports she has needed assistance with self-care and ADLs such as bathing and dressing due to pain and stiffness since her surgery. Pt. & spouse both retired. Pt. states she likes to garden. Pt. is (R) hand dominant.

Patient Goals: Pt. states she wants to return to her normal function.

O: *Palpation:* There is generalized soreness upon palpation of the entire (L) elbow region. Pt. also displays tenderness in the (L) brachioradialis muscle.

Inspection: The pt. displays a well healed incision on the elbow.

ROM: (B) Shoulder AROM WNLs throughout

	(R)	(L)
PROM elbow extension/flexion	0° to 150°	90° to 130°
Forearm supination	90°	45°
Forearm pronation	90°	35°
Wrist flexion	75°	0°
Wrist extension	80°	45°

The patient is unable to make a complete fist with the (L) hand due to discomfort and "stiffness." Formal measurements of finger joints not performed this date due to patient needing to get to a personal function. To be deferred to next session.

Strength: (R) UE 4+/5 to 5/5 throughout all musculature. (L) shoulder 4–/5, (L) elbow pt. unable to tolerate any resistance; does perform against gravity showing 3-/5 of biceps and triceps. Grip strength (R) 40#, (L) 25#.

Intervention: Patient received MHP x 20 mins to (L) elbow and (L) hand. Gentle stretching and mobilization to elbow joints followed this. PT performed AAROM to (L) elbow, wrist and hand 10 repetitions.

Patient Education: The patient was instructed in gentle self ROM techniques. Pt. was issued a written HEP of these ROM activities (see copy in pt. chart). Pt. was advised to use prescription pain medication approximately 30 minutes before the next therapy session to increase tolerance to the activities.

A: The patient displays limited ROM, decreased strength and (L) hand edema, which are impeding her functional tasks at home. The patient had an increase in pain to 6–7/10 during therapeutic ROM and stretching.

STGs: To be achieved within 5 treatment sessions. All impairment goals listed are to facilitate the pt. to be able to be (I) with self-care activities.

1. Decrease edema in the (L) hand to equal the (R)
2. Increase (L) wrist ROM to WNL
3. Increase elbow flexion to 140° and extension to 0°

(continued)

Example 5-8 (continued)

LTGs: To be achieved within 14 treatment sessions. All impairment goals listed are to facilitate pt. to be able to return to normal activities including house work and gardening.

1. Increase strength in the (L) elbow and hand to 4/5 to 4+/5 throughout to allow increased functional activities
2. Increase (L) elbow ROM to WNL to allow normal eating and self-care
3. The patient will be (I) with basic ADLs and IADLs

P: Patient to receive PT 3x/week for modalities, ROM and progressive therapeutic exercises to the (L) elbow, wrist, and hand. Will include general ROM and strengthening exercises to the shoulder to minimize effects of decreased activity on that musculature/joint.

Stephanie Wright, DPT

Chapter 6

Basic Guidelines for Documentation

Rebecca McKnight, PT, MS and Mia L. Erickson, PT, EdD, ATC, CHT

CHAPTER OBJECTIVES

After reading this chapter, the student will be able to do the following:

1. List components of the patient/client management model that should be documented in the medical record.
2. Identify tasks that must be documented by the PT and those that can be documented by the PTA.
3. Describe the purpose of the APTA *Guidelines for Physical Therapy Documentation.*
4. Report basic principles for documentation.
5. Report principles for documenting patient care.
6. Indicate common reasons for denial of payment associated with inappropriate documentation methods.
7. Correctly document late entries and appropriately correct errors in medical records.
8. Follow appropriate guidelines when writing physical therapy notes.

DOCUMENTATION IN PHYSICAL THERAPY

Documentation of physical therapy services occurs over a continuum, throughout a patient's episode of care. Documentation begins with the initial examination, evaluation, and plan of care as performed and written by the PT. Subsequent documentation includes interim notes for every encounter with the patient. Interim notes can be written by either the PT or the PTA. Interim notes are written to record treatment sessions and serve as a record of what was billed. Progress notes are written to reflect the patient's progress toward the goals stated in the initial evaluation. Progress notes are written as the patient's status changes, or within a required time frame as dictated by state law or third-party payers. Final documentation is performed at the summation of care. This is the last entry in a patient's record and is usually referred to as the discharge summary. This note often reflects results of a discharge evaluation, which is also performed and written by the PT. From examination to discharge, the physical therapy record should reflect: (1) the patient's condition, or pathology; (2) impairments and functional deficits identified through appropriate tests and measurements; (3) anticipated goals and expected outcomes; (4) interventions provided, including patient education, communication with other disciplines, and specific procedural interventions; and (5) the final outcome or result of the intervention. It is the position of the APTA that the physical therapy examination, evaluation, diagnosis, and prognosis be documented, dated, and authenticated by the PT performing the service. Interventions provided by the PT or PTA should be documented, dated, and authenticated by the PT, the PTA (where permissible by law), or both.[1] This record should be kept in a secured file to meet confidentiality requirements.

The APTA has set forth standardized *Guidelines for Physical Therapy Documentation of Patient/Client Management.*[1] The purpose of these guidelines is to "provide (documentation) guidance for the physical therapy profession across all practice settings."[1(p703)] Though they are not intended to reflect documentation requirements in all specialty areas, the guidelines can serve as a "foundation" for developing documentation procedures across a variety of unique and specialized settings.[1] Other authors have also reported specific guidelines for documenting in medical records.[2-9]

Erickson M, McKnight R. *Documentation Basics:
A Guide for the Physical Therapist Assistant, Second Edition (pp. 61-72)*
© 2012 SLACK Incorporated

This chapter will discuss basic principles of documentation and will introduce how to structure and how to begin an interim note. Subsequent chapters will provide specific details related to how a PTA will document within the various sections of a SOAP note format.

BASIC PRINCIPLES

- **Be timely**. It is important that documentation is completed as soon after the session as possible. First, the treatment session is fresh in your mind, and you are more likely to remember details sooner after the session rather than later. In addition, your documentation might be necessary so that another therapist or assistant can treat the patient in the event of your absence. There are also managerial reasons for timely documentation. These include filing reimbursement claims and sending progress updates to others involved in the patient's care, including physicians, case managers, or insurance companies. Clinics are likely to have policies in place requiring completion of all patient documentation within a given time frame.
- **Entries must be thorough**. All entries made in the medical record must be relevant, thorough, accurate, and logical. You should be able to examine your records and have an accurate, detailed depiction of the patient and situation. Any clinician should be able to pick up one of your patient records and treat the patient in the case of your absence.
- **Entries must be clear and concise**. Though it is important to be as concise as possible, you should also be thorough. Never leave out pertinent information for the sake of brevity.
- **Be consistent**. Use similar types of documentation throughout the patient's episode of care at your facility (eg, forms, SOAP format, flow sheets). This makes it easy for reviewers and other health care providers to locate necessary information.
- **Use objective language**. Include facts and observations. Avoid making subjective remarks about patients, including anything that cannot be substantiated by the data. This includes subjective remarks about a patient's response to a treatment (eg, "tolerated treatment well"), the patient's personality, or his or her psychological status. Also, avoid subjective terms such as *appears* and *seems to be*.[10] (eg, "Patient seems depressed today"). Though you may be trying to provide additional information about the patient, you must be very careful not to make an unsubstantiated judgment.[7]
- **Write legibly**. Third-party payers have been known to deny claims based solely on the fact that they could not read the provider's handwriting.
- **Use black or blue permanent ink**. Ballpoint is preferred over felt-tip pens. Erasable ink should never be used.
- **Use scientific, medical terminology**. Avoid "nonskilled language" such as "The patient walked. …" Use descriptive, functional language instead, such as "Provided gait and transfer training. …"
- **Entries must communicate skilled care**. Describe how you use your skills to assist the patient. Provide specific language as to how your special skills and training provided assistance to the patient above and beyond what could be provided by an untrained individual. A description of how your skills assisted the patient provides additional insight into the patient's need for skilled services.
  - Example 1: "Facilitated right quadriceps during the swing phase of gait …"
  - Example 2: "Pt. required min (a) x 1 to stabilize (R) knee manually during stance to prevent hyperextension."
- **Use abbreviations appropriately**. Use only industry-standard and facility-approved medical terminology, symbols, and abbreviations (Appendix A). Please note that you should not overuse abbreviations. This can become confusing for the reader, especially if he or she is unfamiliar with any of the abbreviations. In addition, some abbreviations have more than one meaning (eg, PT = physical therapist and prothrombin time). In these cases, you must read the entire note to determine the context of the abbreviation so that you can interpret it appropriately. Check with your facility regarding acceptable abbreviations and their use.
- **Write in the third person**. Use of the first person is generally not acceptable. The third person is preferred because the emphasis should be on what the patient can do or does.
  - Example:
    Instead of: I ambulated the pt. 50' and provided min (A).
    Use: Pt. ambulated 50' c̄ min (A) x 1.
  There are times, however, when the use of first-person language is unavoidable; for example, when there has been a special situation and you are describing what happened in the narrative format.
- **Avoid skipping lines**. When writing in a medical record, you should begin your note with the date of service on the line immediately below the prior entry. Furthermore, you should not skip lines in the middle of your notes. Skipping lines could allow someone to come back at a later date and fraudulently add information.
- **Use headings**. Headings group relevant information together to indicate new sections and to designate important patient information. They often make the note easier to read and identify necessary informa-

tion. You will want to utilize the same headings that were utilized by the PT in the initial evaluation when possible. This will help provide links between the initial evaluation and the interim notes.

- **Use tables when indicated**. In instances where there is a great deal of data that can easily become confusing to the reader, it is appropriate to use tables, columns, or lists. Tables are valuable when documenting range of motion or strength on several joints, such as the hand. See Example 5-7 for an example of the use of tables or columns.

- **Document late entries**. After completing the documentation for a particular treatment session and placing it in the medical record, you might realize a need to document additional information about the session. The original note should never be rewritten. Instead, you should complete a late entry. The entry should be placed in chronological order for the date that it is written and be identified as a "late entry."

  - Late entries. A chart entry is considered a late entry when other health care providers have documented after your original documentation or when enough time has elapsed so that the date on which you are writing the late entry is different from the original documentation. In either case, the entry should be placed in chronological order for the date that it is written and be identified as a late entry. An explanation for the late entry should also be provided.[7]

  - Addendum. An addendum is written immediately following the original documentation. In this case, do not skip a line but identify with the heading: "Addendum." Addendums are usually written because you quickly realize that you have forgotten to write something that should have been included. Sign the addendum as you would your original documentation.

- **Correct errors**. Indicate an error with a single straight black line through the text. An individual reading the note should still be able to read what was written originally. Initial and date next to the error. Never use correction fluid or erasable ink in a medical record.

  - Example: The patient ~~ambulated~~ MLE 2/18/11 transferred with min (A) x 1.

- **Date and authenticate all patient records**. All physical therapy records should be dated according to the day the services were provided. Authentication is "the process used to verify that an entry into the medical record is complete, accurate, and final. Indications of authentication can include original written signatures and computer "signatures" on secured electronic record systems only."[1] Signatures should also include the clinician's full name and designation (PT or PTA).[4]

- **Document missed appointments**. Document reasons for cancelled or missed appointments or treatment sessions whether initiated by the pt., the PT, the PTA, or another health care provider.

  - Example 1:
    In an outpatient clinic, a snow storm in January caused your patient to miss his appointments for 2 days. Document:
    1/19/11—Pt. canceled appt. 2° to weather, rescheduled for 1/21. Sue Brooks, PTA
    1/21/11—Pt. canceled 2° to weather rescheduled for 1/23. Sue Brooks, PTA

  - Example 2:
    On a skilled nursing unit the nurse asks that you not work with a patient because the physician suspects the patient has a DVT and is awaiting a Doppler. Document:
    12/12/11—Attempted to see Mrs. Smith this am; however, nursing asked that we hold therapy 2° to possible DVT, awaiting Doppler. Will resume when cleared. Sue Brooks, PTA

- **Document telephone, face-to-face, or electronic conversations related to patient care**. This could include conversations with the patent, the patient's family, the physician, other health care providers, or case managers. For example, you are working with a 24-year-old who was injured in a workplace accident, and the patient's case manager for workers' compensation contacts you to determine the patient's status and progress. Currently the APTA is investigating the creation of guidelines for any internet consultation.

- **Document unusual or unexpected situations or results**. Some of these situations may also require completion of an incident report. Completion of incident reports will be discussed further in Chapter 11 within the discussion of legal aspects of documentation. For example, you are working with a 22-year-old female who underwent an anterior cruciate ligament (ACL) repair. She is performing resisted knee flexion with a pulley system and felt a "pop" in her knee with a moderate increase in pain.

- **Indicate "continued" when using more than 1 page**. When documentation of patient care requires more than 1 page of entry, make sure that each page includes the patient's name, the patient's medical record number, and the date. You should transition the information by writing a statement like: "PT note for [patient's name and date] continued next page."

TOP 10 REASONS FOR DENIALS FROM PAYERS

APTA's "Defensible documentation" tips sheet records the top 10 payer complaints about documentation that lead to denial of payment for claims. Following the guidelines presented previously will help guard you against several of these reasons for denial.

1. Poor legibility.
2. Incomplete documentation.
3. No documentation for date of service.
4. Abbreviations—too many, cannot understand.
5. Documentation does not support the billing (coding).
6. Does not demonstrate skilled care.
7. Does not support medical necessity.
8. Does not demonstrate progress.
9. Repetitious daily notes showing no change in patient status.
10. Interventions with no clarification of time, frequency, duration.[11]

DOCUMENTING PATIENT CARE

When documenting interventions or services provided in an interim note, you should include specific descriptions of the intervention and equipment provided. This information is frequently documented through the use of checklists, flowcharts, or graphs. To demonstrate the patient's status (progression or regression) you should document the following types of information:

- Subjective information that helps to demonstrate the patient's status.
- Changes in objective and measurable findings as they relate to the initial evaluation and the existing goals.
- The patient's reaction to treatment (positive or negative).
- Progression/regression of the treatment plan, including patient education.
- Communication or collaboration with other health care providers, the patient, and the patient's family or caregiver(s).[1]

Each interim note needs to both refer to the initial evaluation and be able to stand alone. The information documented in an interim note helps to demonstrate progression of therapy services, as well as the patient's response to those services, so the note needs to be structured to demonstrate how the information refers to the initial plan of care. On the other hand, each note needs to be written as clearly as possible and with enough detail that it can independently support the intervention provided that day (Table 6-1).

REFERENCES

1. American Physical Therapy Association. Guidelines: Physical Therapy Documentation of Patient/Client Management. G03-05-16-41. Available at: http:www.apta.org/uploadedFiles/APTAorg/About_Us/Policies/BOD/Practice/DocumentationPatientClientMgamt.pdf. Accessed May 24, 2011.
2. Redgate N, Foto M. Pay by the rules: avoid Medicare audits and reduce payment denials with a sound strategy and proper documentation. *Physical Therapy Products.* October/November 2003:28–30.
3. Inaba M, Jones SL. Medical documentation for third-party payers. *Phys Ther.* 1977;57:791–794.
4. Goode N. The reliable resource: physical therapy documentation. *PT Magazine.* 1999;7(9):30–31.
5. Arriaga R. Liability awareness. Stories from the front: documentation and clinical decision making: a real-life scenario illustrates some basic risk-management principles. *PT Magazine.* 2002;10(5):46–49.
6. Lewis K. Do the write thing: document everything. *PT Magazine.* 2002;10(7):30–34.
7. Schunk CR. Liability awareness. Advice for the new physical therapist: here are some keys to avoiding risk once you've made the transition from student to practitioner. *PT Magazine.* 2001;9(11):24–26.
8. White JA. Managing care. Documentation: making it meaningful. *Physical Therapy Case Reports.* 2000;3(2):78–79.
9. Abeln SH. Liability awareness. Reporting risk check-up. *PT Magazine.* 1997;5(10):38–42.
10. Clifton DW Jr. "Tolerated treatment well" may no longer be tolerated. *PT Magazine.* 1995;3(10):24.
11. American Physical Therapy Association. Defensible documentation for patient/client management. Available at: http://www.apta.org/Documentation/DefensibleDocumentation. Accessed February 1, 2012.

Table 6-1

INFORMATION FOUND IN AN INITIAL EVALUATIVE NOTE COMPARED TO AN INTERIM NOTE IN THE SOAP FORMAT

Initial Evaluation		Interim Note

• Patient's chief complaint
• Medical diagnosis
• Physical therapy diagnosis
• Loss of function
• Any information gleaned from the medical record
   o Recent or past surgeries
   o Past conditions or diseases
   o Present conditions or diseases
   o Results of medical tests
	Pr:	• Patient's chief complaint
		• Medical diagnosis
		• Physical therapy diagnosis
		• Loss of function
		• New test results

• Patient's current and past medical history • Patient's symptoms or complaints • Factors that cause the symptoms or complaints • Patient's prior level of function • Patient's lifestyle/occupation/societal roles • Patient's goals	S:	• Patient's status • Patient's reaction to intervention • New problems or new complaints • Pertinent information not previously documented

• Information gathered through
   o Tests
   o Measures
   o Observation
• Interventions provided
• Patient's response to interventions provided
• Patient education
	O:	• Patient status
		   o Data collected
		   o Patient's functional status
		   o Observations
		• Interventions provided
		   o Communication/collaboration
		   o Patient-related instruction
		   o Procedural interventions

• Physical therapist's interpretation of the S and O data • Identification of impairments and functional limitations • Goals • Physical therapy diagnosis • Prognosis/rehabilitation potential • Justification for goals/treatment plan • Explanation of any difficulties with obtaining S or O data • Suggestions for further testing, treatment, or referrals	A:	• A summarization of the S and O data • Response to interventions • Reference to how the patient is progressing toward the goals established in the plan of care

• Plan for intervention activities to occur
   o Collaboration/communication
   o Patient-related education
   o Procedural interventions
• Frequency/duration of therapy services
• Treatment progression
• Plans for further assessment or reassessment
• Equipment needs
• Referral to other services
	P:	• What actions need to occur within areas of intervention
		   o Communication/collaboration
		   o Patient-related instruction
		   o Procedural interventions
		• When the next session is scheduled
		• Any equipment or information that needs to be ordered or prepared before the next session

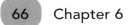

Review Questions

1.   Who is responsible for writing the initial examination? Interim notes? Progress notes? Discharge summaries?

2.   What is the purpose of the *Guidelines for Physical Therapy Documentation?*

3.   How much time should elapse between treating a patient and documenting the session?

4.   What color inks are most appropriate for medical record documentation?

5.   What does the term *authenticate* mean?

APPLICATION EXERCISES

I. For the following entries, indicate examples that are inappropriate by writing an *I* next to the item. Describe why they are inappropriate.

_____ The patient walked 50'.

_____ Skilled services are needed.

_____ Pt. stated that she enjoys coming to PT.

_____ Pt. c/o pain in the (L) knee following exercise p̄ last visit.

_____ AROM: (R) shoulder flexion 160° abduction 120°.

_____ Pt. performed QS, GS, and SLRs.

_____ Pt. walked around the PT gym 2x.

_____ ROM knee 0–135°.

_____ Pt. demonstrating global aphasia.

_____ Pt. is demonstrating excessive hip abduction c̄ his prosthesis during ambulation.

_____ Gait: 100' c̄ hemi-walker c̄ min (A) x 1 for trunk support and min (A) x 1 for advancing the (L) LE.

_____ Transfers: Bed ↔ chair c̄ min (A) x 1 2° to poor balance.

_____ Ther Ex: Performed 20 repetitions all exercises.

_____ Bed mobility: Rolls supine ↔ SL with min (A) x 1.

_____ HEP: Instructed the pt. in a HEP to be performed tid.

II. Write the following information in a more clear and concise manner, as it would appear in the medical record.

1. The patient walked 75 feet in the hallway of the hospital with the therapist lightly touching her back. She used a front-wheeled walker.

2. The patient's strength was 3/5 for the right biceps and 4/5 for the right triceps.

3. Upon arrival to therapy, the patient told you that she had been doing her HEP without any problems and really felt like her ability to get in and out of bed had improved.

4. The patient said that her pain was 3/10 on a pain scale.

5. You performed ultrasound to the dorsal aspect of the patient's right foot. You used 3 MHz at 50% duty cycle with the intensity set at 1.0 w/cm^2.

6. The patient demonstrated the following range of motion measurements: active range of motion for the right elbow was 130° flexion and 10° of hyperextension.

7. Knee active range of motion was 100° flexion and lacking 10° of extension.

8. The patient propelled his wheelchair around the hospital, outside on the sidewalk, and up and down several ramps with you providing verbal reminders on trunk positioning for going up and down the ramps.

9. The patient was able to put her ankle–foot orthosis on and remove it independently. She was also able to independently check her skin for any irritated areas after she removed the orthosis.

10. You instructed the patient to perform 10 repetitions of each exercise as part of her home exercise program. The exercises included ankle pumps, quadriceps setting, short arc quadriceps strengthening from 45° to 0°, and heel slides.

11. During a busy morning in a hospital, you were working with a patient who told you that she was going to be discharged and wanted home health services, primarily PT. After writing the note and moving on to the next patient, you realize that you did not document the patient's desire for home PT. What should you do? In the space below, demonstrate how you would document this entry into the chart? Where should this information be placed?

12. When writing the following information in the chart, you realize that you made an error in documenting the patient's AROM. It should have been 125°, not 152°. Demonstrate how to correct this mistake.

III. Organize the following information so that it is clear, concise, and suitable for entry into the medical record.
1. Mr. Jones comes into the clinic today and tells you that his fingers became swollen and that he has had pain at a level of 7 out of 10 since the last treatment session. He goes on to say that he has not been able to perform any of the range of motion exercises you gave him because of the incredible amount of pain he has been having. He said that he has changed his postoperative dressing once a day, and he has had a little bit of red drainage on the bandages. He also said that he is having trouble eating and shaving due to the swelling and stiffness in the joints.

2. You enter Mrs. Smith's hospital room and ask her if she is ready for treatment. She agrees and tells you that she wants to be ready to walk down the aisle at her grandson's wedding without using her walker. She said that her right knee pain is not as bad as it was yesterday and she thinks that she is able to bend it more. She goes on to say that she has performed the range of motion exercises twice already this morning, and she is working on trying to get her knee to bend as much as she can. While walking, she asks if she can begin using a cane soon.

3. Mr. Smith comes into the Physical Therapy Department and tells you that he notices improvement in his walking since beginning the active range of motion exercises for his ankle. He also says that he is having 0 out of 10 pains with the new exercises. He goes on to tell you that he still has pain when walking on gravel, carpet, and stairs. His job (logger) requires him to do a lot of walking on uneven terrain, and he wants to be able to do this without pain before returning to work.

4. You are assigned an inpatient who had a right cerebral vascular accident 3 weeks ago. The supervising PT told you that she is demonstrating confusion and slurred speech, but her daughter is usually present during the sessions. Upon entering the patient's room, you notice that the daughter is not present. As you work with the patient, she tells you that she fell in the bathroom last night. She also tells you that she is afraid to get out of

bed because of her fear of falling again. It was difficult for you to understand the patient due to the slurring. You also understand the patient to say that her left shoulder is sore. While performing bedside active assistive range of motion, her daughter returns, and you comment to the daughter about the patient's fall the previous night. The daughter tells you that there wasn't a fall and that she had been there with her mother all night.

5. While treating a patient during a home health visit, the patient's son tells you that his mother (the patient) has been up all night due to left hip pain. He also tells you that he is having trouble getting his mother to walk in the house with him due to pain and fear of making her hip hurt more than it already does. He also says that he has trouble performing the range of motion exercises that you showed him during the last session. The patient tells you that, because of the pain, she feels like her hip is going to give out when she stands on it.

6. Passive range of motion measurements were as follows: Right knee flexion 100°, right knee extension 5°, hip abduction 20°, hip flexion 100°, ankle PF 20°, elbow 10–100°, shoulder flexion 100°, shoulder abduction 100°, hip IR 20°, ankle DF 5°, shoulder ER 60°, and IR 45°.

7. Walked 10', twice, with one person supplying 25% assistance, used a standard walker, did not put any weight on the right leg, needed verbal reminders each time for placing the walker forward.

8. Up and down 4 stairs with a handrail that was on the right side going up and on the left coming down; the patient used a straight cane. He required supervision from the PTA.

9. The patient walked with the therapist at his side (but not touching him) for 100 feet, twice; vital signs before exercise were blood pressure 125/85, 15 for respirations, and 77 for heart rate; vitals after were 135/85 for blood pressure, 17 for respirations, and 87 for heart rate; the patient performed ankle pumping, elbow flexion, shoulder flexion, and knee extension for 10 repetitions before and after exercise.

10. Girth at the right knee joint line was 34 cm, 2 inches above was 38 cm, 4 inches above was 42 cm, and 4 inches below was 35.5 cm. Active flexion was 120°. The patient lacked 20° of active extension. Hip and ankle active range of motion were within normal limits. Strength for the quadriceps muscle was 3–/5 and for the hamstring was 3–/5. The patient walks independently with crutches, weight bearing as much as he can tolerate on the involved extremity for 100 feet.

11. You are working with a patient with a diagnosis of bicipital tendonitis in an outpatient clinic. She tells you that she has been working on the home exercises and, overall, her arm is feeling much better. She reports pain to be 3/10 on a verbal pain scale. She says that she has trouble reaching into overhead cabinets and shelves. Her treatment consisted of ultrasound over the anterior shoulder for 6 minutes, 50% duty cycle, with the intensity set at 1.5 w/cm^2. This was followed by gentle active range of motion exercises with a wand for flexion and external rotation, active scapular retraction and protraction, prone horizontal abduction, and external rotation with yellow exercise band for 2 sets of 10 repetitions. She also received manual stretching for flexion, internal rotation, and external rotation (performed by you). The treatment concluded with ice for 15 minutes. She reported better range of motion and less pain when the treatment was over. She will return 2 times each week for the above treatment and progression of the exercises as tolerated.

12. You are working with a patient 3 days status post-right total knee replacement in the PT gym. She has noticeable swelling and limited range of motion in the knee and ankle. She transfers to and from the mat with you providing 25% assistance. She transferred sit to and from supine with you performing 50% assistance due to her inability to lift the right leg onto the mat table. She performed 2 sets of 10 repetitions of the total knee exercises and ambulated 50 feet, twice, with a standard walker, only putting 50% of her body weight on the involved extremity. She received ice for 15 minutes to her knee. You notice that she walked only 25' during yesterday's session. She will be seen in the afternoon for the same treatment, progressing gait as tolerated.

IV. Organize the following information so that it is clear, concise, and suitable for entry into the medical record. Use the initial evaluative note (Example 6-1) when writing the note.

1. You have treated the patient today (December 6, 2010) and note the following. Write a progress note based upon this information.

When you enter the room the patient is finishing with his bathing. The nurse helps him to dress in his jogging pants and sweatshirt. You ask if he is ready for therapy. He grumbles a bit but agrees. The patient seems irritated. Upon inquiry he reports that he wants to go home but "you guys won't let me." You respond appropriately to that statement. You assist the patient to the therapy department. Given the choice of whether to walk first or exercise first the patient chooses to walk. The patient is sitting on the edge of the bed and has no trouble standing up to his walker. You help the patient walk. He tires after about 75 feet but he is able to walk with only verbal cues for using his walker appropriately. After the patient takes a brief rest break in a chair, you help him practice ambulating on stairs. The patient has difficulty with the task and needs 25% assistance for walker placement and a boost to raise himself up the steps. He states that his shoulders are hurting and that going up the stairs really bothers them. You assist the patient to the therapy mat where he needs assistance to raise his operated limb up onto the mat while lying down. The patient performs all the exercises the therapist previously ordered—2 sets of 10 repetitions each. The patient still required assistance with straight-leg raises. The therapist also had asked you to add shoulder exercises. The patient performed all shoulder movements with a 2-pound weight for 1 set of 10 repetitions. After the mat exercises, you have the patient sit up. He needs a little bit of physical assistance to get his leg off the mat and to help push up his upper body. You then help him to perform standing hip extension, flexion, and abduction of his affected limb while holding onto his walker. You assist the patient back to his chair and back to his room, telling him you will be back for another session in the afternoon.

Example 6-1

Anytown Community Hospital: Skilled Nursing Facility

Physical Therapy Evaluation
Patient: I.H.
Age: 67 y.o.
Date: 12/03/10
Referral: Physical therapy for gait and strengthening. Anterior hip precautions, WBAT
Referring Physician: Dr. Mark John
Pr: Pain and DJD (L) Hip s/p THA
Hx: This 67-y.o. patient was admitted for a THA 11/30/10. PMH includes DJD bilateral shoulders, HTN and 2 previous TIAs approx. 1 year ago.
S: *Complaint:* The patient states he does have general soreness but his hip pain is less than before the surgery. Rates pain as 1–2/10.
Living Environment/Social Support: The patient lives at home with spouse. Has 3 steps with railing to enter his one-level home. The patient states his hobbies include yard work and doing crossword puzzles.
Prior Level of Function/Activities: The patient was previously (I) with shoulder level and below ADLs and gait without (A) device.
Goals: The patient wants to return to his normal level of functioning.

O: ROM

		(L)	(R)
Hip			
	Flexion	0 to 30	0 to 135
	Abduction	0	0 to 30
Shoulder			
	Flexion	0 to 90	0 to 95
	Abduction	0 to 75	0 to 80

Peripheral Vascular Assessment:

		(L)	(R)
Color		Slight pallor; refill brisk	Pink
Temp		Toes slightly cool	Warm
Touch		Intact	Intact
Pulses			
	Dorsalis pedis	Regular; slight diminished	Regular and full

Girth: (L) 3 cm > (R); 8 cm at the center of the patella
Strength: 4/5 to 4+/5 throughout (B) UE's and (R) LE except shoulders 3+/5. (L) hip MMT deferred 2° to recent surgery; appears 2/5 with functional mobility. (L) knee strength 3+/5, ankle strength 5/5.
Mobility: Scooting in bed with min (A) x 1, supine ↔ sit with mod (A) x 1, sit ↔ stand with min (A) x 1.
Gait: Pt. ambulated 50' with walker and min (A) x 1 WBAT (L) LE. Pt. needed frequent v/cs for proper walker placement. Pt. had a tendency to place walker too far in front of him. c/o mild discomfort in shoulders with using walker.
Intervention: Initiated AAROM to (L) LE. Pt. performed ankle pumps, quad sets, ham sets, glut sets, SAQ, SLR, hip abd, and heel slides 1 x 10.
Pt. Education: Pt. was instructed in hip precautions and was given a written reminder sheet of precautions.
A: Pt. is very motivated and has excellent rehab potential. Extremity segment, peripheral vascular check, and ROM all within post-THA limits.
Problem List:
1. Decreased strength (L) LE
2. Dependent mobility
3. Dependent gait
4. Hip precautions

STGs: To be met within 2 days
1. Increase (L) LE strength to 3–/5 throughout hip and 3+/5 knee to allow normal functional mobility.
2. Pt. will require SBA-CGA x 1 with all bed mobility & transfers.
3. Pt. will ambulate 100' c̄ walker & CGA x 1 on level surfaces.
4. Pt. will be able to verbalize hip precautions.

(continued)

Example 6-1 (continued)

LTGs: To be met within 7 days
1. Increase (L) LE strength to 3+/5 throughout hip and 4/5 knee to allow normal functional mobility.
2. Pt. will be (I) c̄ all bed mobility & transfers.
3. Pt. will ambulate 200' c̄ walker (I) on level surface & up and down 3 steps with SBA x 1.
4. Pt. will display good understanding of hip precautions during all functional activities.

P: PT BID for transfer and gait training, ROM/strengthening exercises, and education regarding hip precautions.

Mary Good, DPT

Chapter 7

Writing the Subjective Section

Rebecca McKnight, PT, MS

CHAPTER OBJECTIVES

After reading this chapter, the student will be able to do the following:

1. List sources of information for subjective (history) data.
2. Identify types of data that should be recorded in the subjective portion of a SOAP note.
3. Discuss how subjective data are used to inform the clinical decision-making process.
4. List types of information that should be recorded in the subjection section of the interim note.
5. Describe the importance of linking subjective information in the interim note with information in the evaluative note.

INTRODUCTION

Subjective data is information that the PTA gleans through ways other than through direct observation. *Webster's Dictionary* defines *subjective* as "characteristic of or belonging to reality as perceived rather than as independent of mind," "peculiar to a particular individual," "modified or affected by personal views, experience, or background," and "lacking in reality or substance."[1] These definitions imply that subjective information may be lacking in validity or reliability due to the personal perspectives attained. As a PTA, you need to keep in mind that subjective data gathered from the patient (or other individuals) does in fact carry that individual's personal perspective, and this perspective has great bearing on how the patient will respond to therapeutic interventions.

WHERE DOES IT COME FROM?

In most cases, subjective information is data gathered from the patient through direct and specific questioning. Individuals who are in close relationships with the patient may also be able to provide direct information about the patient's condition and functional status. The patient's family or caregiver can provide additional information and alternate perspectives that can help form a more comprehensive view of the patient's status. In cases where the patient has cognitive or communicative limitations and where no medical records exist, the subjective information may come entirely from the family or caregiver. In these situations, the PTA should identify the individual who has the closest contact with the patient. This person will likely be the individual who can provide the clearest picture of the patient's functional abilities and limitations.

Subjective information includes data that provide insight into the patient's condition and its impact on the patient's functional mobility and activity participation. The PTA should remain alert to patient and caregiver comments related to the impairments in body functions, functional limitations, and activity restrictions associated to the current condition. This information will also help the physical therapist assistant discern the patient's affective response to these issues and will allow the PTA to respond appropriately or modify the intervention strategies as necessary. Specific statements that provide a view into the patient's perspective and functional status should be quoted within the interim note. Subjective information can provide a view into the psychosocial issues and contextual factors that influence the patient's functioning and participation.

Erickson M, McKnight R. *Documentation Basics: A Guide for the Physical Therapist Assistant, Second Edition (pp. 73-78)*

The subjective section of the SOAP note answers the question, "What does the patient (or the patient's family member/caregiver) have to say?" The subjective information provides the patient's perspective and documents valuable information to support the effectiveness of the treatment plan or demonstrate the need for alteration of the treatment plan. When writing the S section, you will document any comments from the patient or the patient's family member(s), caregiver(s), or significant other(s) that demonstrate (1) the patient's status/progress, (2) the patient's reaction to interventions provided, or (3) new problems or complaints or any pertinent information not previously documented.

PROBLEM (PR)

You will need to record the problem prior to recording the subjective information. The problem section of the SOAP note answers the question, "What is the main problem?" In an interim note you should document the diagnosis or main physical therapy problem. This information helps to provide a context for the rest of the documentation. You can find this information in the initial evaluation. In this section you may also include results of any new tests or procedures from the medical record such as radiographs or lab results (Example 7-1).

SUBJECTIVE (S)

After recording the problem, you can begin to record the subjective information. The following are examples of subjective information you might need to include in the interim note.

Patient's Status

- **Pain rating and description.** For example, a 48-year-old male, who is recovering from a back injury, was asked to rate his pain using a numerical scale of 0 to 10 (0 = *no pain* and 10 = *worst possible pain*). The patient currently rates his pain as 3/10 and describes the pain as a "pulling" pain.
- **Patient's perception of symptoms.** For example, a 76-year-old male in a skilled nursing facility who is recovering from an exacerbation of chronic obstructive pulmonary disease (COPD), reports, "I am feeling stronger."
- **Patient's functional abilities.** For example, a 35-year-old female recovering from complications resulting from a radical mastectomy reports, "I was able to put the dishes into the cabinet last night for the first time since my surgery."
- **Statements that demonstrate the patient's cognitive or emotional status.** For example, an 84-year-old female, recovering from an open reduction internal

---

Example 7-1

Anytown Community Hospital: Skilled Nursing Facility

Physical Therapy Progress Note
Patient: D.T.
Date: 04/04/11
Pr: Left patellectomy; (L) LE ROM & strength deficits

---

fixation (ORIF) of a fractured femur, has been a widow for several years and was living alone prior to the accident. While in therapy, the patient comments that her husband is waiting in her room to take her dancing.

- **Comments related to accomplishment of goals/outcomes.** For example, you are working with a 32-year-old female who is recovering from a humeral fracture. One of her personal goals is to be able to care for her 10-month-old infant. Today, in the clinic, she proudly reports, "I was able to change the baby's diaper last night all by myself."

Informed Consent

- Informed consent is a method of informing the patient of the treatment or care that you will be providing. Initially, the PT obtains informed consent when discussing the plan of care with the patient. However, you might be required to obtain informed consent when implementing a new modality. In this case, you are required to explain the procedure, determine the presence of contraindications, and describe risks and benefits where appropriate. You will want to record the patient's consent to the new intervention in the subjective area of the interim note.

Patient's Response to Interventions Provided

- **Behavior of the patient's pain since the previous intervention.** For example, a 52-year-old female is receiving therapy due to a diagnosis of adhesive capsulitis. The patient states that her pain level increased after her last therapy session when a new stretching activity was initiated, but she reports the increase in pain only lasted about 1 hour and then the pain returned to its normal level.
- **Comments that demonstrate whether the intervention provided is effective.** For example, a 64-year-old male suffering from chronic cervical pain has received a trial of transcutaneous electrical nerve stimulation (TENS). The patient reports no relief of pain symptoms with the TENS trial.

Example 7-2

S: Pt. c/o continued weakness in (L) knee. Reports being ambulatory with no assistive device when at home, uses one crutch when on uneven surfaces, outside of the home. States he has made moderate improvements with therapy.

New Problem(s) or New Complaint(s)

- **New pain complaints**. For example, a 77-year-old male patient is recovering from an elective total hip arthroplasty (THA). The patient had medical complications and was on bed rest longer than anticipated, and his recovery has been delayed. As you begin working with him, he comments that his heels have been very sore from lying on the bed so much.

Pertinent Information Not Previously Documented

- **Medical history**. For example, you are working in an outpatient setting. You have been assisting with the care of a 48-year-old male who injured his back while moving. Today, as you are working with him, he informs you that he had a hernia repair 2 years ago. You know that this information was not included in the initial evaluation or any of the subsequent interim notes.
- **Environment: lifestyle, home situation, work, school**. For example, you have been assisting with the care of a 72-year-old man in a skilled nursing facility. He had a femur fracture and will be non-weight-bearing (NWB) for 6 to 8 weeks per the physician's report. The patient's goal is to return home, where he lives alone. You know from the evaluative note that the patient has 4 steps without any railing to enter his home. As you are working with the patient he reveals that his "steps" are nothing more than cinder blocks stacked on top of each other.

Structure/Organization

The subjective data are often highly organized in the initial evaluative note. The PT will often categorize information under subheadings to provide structure to the note and to allow for a logical flow of the information. Subheadings for the information can vary and may be delineated by facility policy. When writing an interim note, subheadings are not generally necessary. You will want to organize the subjective information by grouping similar information. You will want to keep all information related to the patient's pain (rating, description, and behavior) together and keep all information related to the home environment (distance needed to walk, steps to negotiate, type of flooring) together. There may be a few occasions when you will need to document many pieces of subjective information. In this case, you can use subheadings to organize the information. When possible, use the same subheadings used by the PT in the initial evaluation. Subheadings that might be used in the subjective section include:

- Current condition
- Patient complaint(s)
- Living environment
- Functional status/activity level
- Medical/surgical history
- Family health history
- Social history
- Employment status

Tips

When writing the subjective information:

- Indicate exactly who is providing the information; for example, the patient, the patient's spouse, the patient's son or daughter, the caregiver.
- Use verbs like *states, reports, complains of, denies, describes*, etc.
- Use quotes to demonstrate the patient's cognitive or emotional status or attitude toward therapy.
- While the first word of the subjective is usually *Pt.* it is not necessary to repeat Pt. at the beginning of every sentence. Once it is written the first time, it is implied in subsequent sentences (Example 7-2).[2]

REFERENCES

1. Merriam-Webster's online dictionary. Subjective. Available at: http://www.m-w.com/dictionary/subjective. Accessed November 13, 2006.
2. Kettenbach G. *Writing SOAP Notes*. 2nd ed. Philadelphia, Pa: F.A. Davis; 1995.

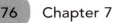

REVIEW QUESTIONS

1. Describe the types of information that should be documented in the subjective portion of an interim SOAP note.

2. Identify appropriate sources for obtaining subjective information. Compare and contrast the validity of each source.

3. Indicate the preferred source (patient, patient's family member/caregiver, patient's medical chart) to obtain the following information and describe why that is the preferred source.

   _____ Number of steps leading into the home

   _____ Description of pain

   _____ Patient's ability to get in/out of bed

   _____ Patient's prior health status

   _____ Last time pain medication was taken

   _____ Sleep patterns

   _____ Patient's adjustment to a permanent disability

   _____ Distance from the bed to the bathroom

   _____ School-related expectations for a pediatric client

APPLICATION EXERCISES

I.   Write the following statements in a more clear and concise manner, as it would appear in the medical record. Indicate the subheading that the information would fall under.

1.   The patient said that his global functional rating is 85% on a 100-point scale.

2.   The patient said he is planning to return home after he is released from the hospital.

3.   The patient's wife said that the patient has not been able to get up out of bed by himself for the past 2 weeks.

4.   The patient said he has not been able to complete his work tasks because he gets tired and has to sit down about every 5 minutes.

5.   The patient's husband tells the PTA that to get from the car to the house the patient will have to walk about 25 feet over grass and then will need to go up 4 steps and that the steps do not have a railing.

II.   Organize the following information so that it is clear, concise, and suitable for entry into the medical record.

1.   You are working with Mr. Jones, who injured his hand in a work accident. He complains of continued swelling in his fingers. He says that he has pain at a level of 7 out of 10 on a 10-point scale. He says he has not been able to make a fist and has had difficulty with getting dressed and eating due to the swelling and pain in his hand.

2.   Upon seeing a child for a school-based intervention, the teacher tells you that she noticed a red spot on the arch of the child's right foot after removing his "leg brace" (a rigid ankle-foot orthosis). She also tells you the child is refusing to walk in the classroom and doesn't put weight on the right foot when transferring in or out of his wheelchair.

3.   You are seeing a 2-year-old girl in the state's early intervention program. She has a congenital right transtibial amputation. She is in foster care. During the session, the foster mom tells you that the child will be getting fit for a new prosthesis and that her doctor recommended she go to a rehabilitation hospital to learn how to use it.

4.   A 19-year-old patient is in a coma after a motor vehicle accident. The patient's mother states that the patient is a very active individual and is involved in basketball and baseball. The mother says that the patient was attending college at the local university and has been living in the dorm rooms. The mother states that the patient has been responding to her by squeezing her hand but that the patient has not said anything to her.

Chapter 8

Writing the Objective Section

Rebecca McKnight, PT, MS

CHAPTER OBJECTIVES

After reading this chapter, the student will be able to do the following:

1. Identify types of data that should be recorded in the objective portion of a SOAP note.
2. Discuss how objective data are used to inform the decision related to provision of patient care.
3. Arrange data collected during the objective portion of an interim note into a logically sequenced, objective note.
4. Describe the importance of linking objective information in the interim note with information in the evaluative note.

INTRODUCTION

The objective section of a SOAP note answers the questions, "What is going on with the physical therapy intervention?" and "How is the patient responding to the intervention?" Objective data include information obtained through various methods and techniques such as range of motion measurements, gross muscle testing, sensation testing, girth measurements, and functional tests. When possible, these methods are based on clearly defined procedures and are therefore reproducible. Using reproducible methods helps to improve the validity and reliability of the data obtained. These measurements are used as baseline

data to which all future data are compared to determine the patient's response(s) to intervention(s). Because objective data are gathered through reproducible procedures, the information is verifiable and therefore useful for validating the need for physical therapy services. Objective data are the information that future measurements can be compared to in order to demonstrate the patient's progress throughout the episode of care. Objective data are used to form a detailed picture of the patient and the problem(s) and are used to guide the physical therapy decision-making process. It is important to remember that the primary goal of physical therapy should be to impact the individual at the activity or participation levels. Documentation of objective data should indicate how the patient's function has been affected. Documentation of function is imperative within current practice guidelines. Reimbursement is typically tied to improvement in function; thus, documentation of limitations in a patient's functional abilities helps to justify the need for physical therapy services. A focus on function also helps with patient motivation because functional activities are more meaningful to patients. For example, a patient is not as interested in how many degrees of motion she has available in her shoulder joint except in how it correlates with her ability to comb her hair.

THE INTERIM NOTE

Objective information in an interim note falls into 1 of 3 categories: (1) physical therapy intervention provided,

Erickson M, McKnight R. *Documentation Basics:*
A Guide for the Physical Therapist Assistant, Second Edition (pp. 79-90)

(2) information that demonstrates the patient's readiness to participate with physical therapy, or (3) information that demonstrates the patient's response to the physical therapy intervention provided.

INTERVENTION PROVIDED

- **Communication and coordination**; for example, discussion with nursing staff about the patient's pain medication schedule.
- **Patient-related instruction**; for example, education related to hip precautions with a patient who is recovering from a THA.
- **Procedural interventions**; for example, transfer and gait training, therapeutic exercise program, physical agents.

DATA THAT INDICATE THAT IT IS SAFE FOR THE PATIENT TO PARTICIPATE IN THE SELECTED INTERVENTIONS

- **Cardiovascular status**. Must include resting heart rate and blood pressure readings.
- **Other data**. May also include various other data collected by the PTA or notes from the medical chart (eg, lab values).

PATIENT'S RESPONSE TO PHYSICAL THERAPY INTERVENTION PROVIDED

Responses are demonstrated by the following:
- **Data collected**. The results of all data collection techniques such as goniometry or manual muscle testing.
- **Description of the patient's function**. For example, description of the patient's ability to move around in bed.
- **Observations about the patient**. Any general observations that cannot be categorized as data from a specific technique or a description of function. This may include information such as description of an open wound, description of patient's movement strategies, or documentation of tenderness to palpation.

STRUCTURE/ORGANIZATION OF O

There is no strict standard structure for documentation of objective data. However, the information should be presented in a logical sequence in order to assist the clinical decision-making process of all involved in patient care and to allow reviewers of the documentation to be able to determine the physical therapist's clinical reasoning process. To allow for easy identification of data, it is necessary to organize the information with the use of subheadings. You should refer to the initial evaluation to determine which subheadings to utilize. This will allow individuals to find information quickly and easily and will help to demonstrate the patient's progress toward the established goals. In addition, when documenting interventions that have been provided, it is important to clearly distinguish the intervention data from the tests and measurement data. This can be accomplished by separating tests and measurement data from the interventions data and by clearly labeling the interventions as such. When you have information that does not easily fall within the subheadings noted in the initial evaluative note, you may choose alternative subheadings. Appropriate subheadings for the objective portion of the note are as follows:
- Aerobic capacity
- Anthropometric characteristics (ie, girth)
- Arousal, attention, and cognition
- Balance
- Circulation (ie, vitals—heart rate and blood pressure, pulses, capillary refill)
- Cranial and peripheral nerve integrity
- Environmental, home, and work barriers
- Ergonomics and body mechanics
- Gait
- Integumentary integrity
- Joint integrity or mobility
- Locomotion (moving from one place to another; ie, transfers)
- Motor function
- Muscle performance (ie, strength, power, and endurance)
- Neuromotor development and sensory integration
- Orthotic, protective, and supportive devices
- Pain (although verbally stated pain and global ratings are indicated in the subjective portion of the note; eg, Pain Numerical Rating Scales and Pain Verbal Rating Scales)
- Posture
- Prosthetic devices
- Range of motion (active range of motion [AROM], passive range of motion [PROM], and flexibility)
- Reflexes
- Self-care and home management skills
- Sensation
- Ventilation/respiration
- Work, community, or leisure status and integration or reintegration (including IADL)

For a thorough description of each of these, including definitions and tools used for gathering data, see the *Guide for Physical Therapist Practice*.[1]

Often information in the objective section is best communicated in list, column, or table format. These formats are used to make the information easier to follow. Columns or tables are also used to document comparative data, such as previous status compared to current status or preintervention measurements compared to postintervention measurements. Information that is frequently documented in this format includes goniometric and manual muscle test results.

Example:

	AROM	PROM	Strength
(R) Hip Abduction	20°	30°	2-/5
Adduction	0°	10°	2-/5
Flexion	80°	95°	3-/5
Extension	0°	5°	2+/5
(R) Knee	10-100°	5-120°	3-/5
(R) Ankle DF	5°	20°	3-/5
PF	45°	45°	4/5
Inv	20°	30°	3+/5
Ev	5°	15°	3+/5

GENERAL TIPS

- When documenting results of tests and measures, it is important that all pertinent information be included to allow for reproduction of the test. Standard testing procedures will be assumed; therefore, if any alterations to the procedure are used, these should be clearly detailed.
- Document results of tests and measures in the same manner as they were performed and documented in the PT's initial evaluative note. Use the same scale used in the initial evaluation.
- All data should be recorded in relationship to what the patient did, not what the PTA did. For example, when documenting gait the note would read:
  - ○ Gait: Pt. ambulated 100' with a straight cane on level surfaces requiring mod (A) x 1, not Gait: The PT walked the patient 100' providing mod (A).
- As with subjective data, complete sentences are not a requirement as in the above example. However, all pertinent information needs to be included.
- Not all information addressed in the initial evaluation needs to be addressed in each interim note.
  - ○ Only address data obtained while reassessing the patient during the treatment session.
  - ○ It is not necessary to address areas that were found to be within normal parameters in the initial examination/evaluation if those areas are still normal.
- A copy of any written instructions provided to the

Example 8-1

O: *AROM* (L) knee   <u>Pretreatment</u>   <u>Post-treatment</u>
      Flex   0° to 135°   0° to 140°
Strength: (L) LE quads 3+/5, hamstrings 4−/5, mild discomfort noticed with knee extension
Gait: Able to ambulate 250' without assistive device or immobilizer independently but does display decreased cadence and guarding. Demonstrates abnormal heel → toe gait pattern and has a tendency to keep LE extended when walking.
Treatment: (L) LE ham curls prone 2 x 10, 5#, LAQs 2 x 10 1#, SLR 2 x 10 no weight. Initiated closed chain knee (B) bends for proprioceptive retraining 3 x 30.

patient should be included in the medical record and referred to in the O section of the note.
- Use verbs like *demonstrated, performed, appears, is,* etc.

TIPS FOR DOCUMENTING INTERVENTIONS PROVIDED

When documenting interventions provided, include all information that is necessary to reproduce the activity (Example 8-1):

- **Intervention provided.** Specify what intervention was provided; for example, modality, exercise, or gait training
- **Intervention amount.** Indicate the dosage or amount of the intervention provided; for example, number of repetitions or distance covered
- **Equipment used.** Indicate any equipment used during the intervention; for example, TENS, 5-lb weight, standard walker
- **Settings.** Provide the setting used with the equipment; for example, ramp on/off time with electrical modalities or pounds of traction
- **Treatment area.** Indicate the specific area of the patient's body that was treated; for example, (L) biceps, insertion of the (R) deltoid
- **Patient positioning.** Specify patient positioning used during the session unless it is a standard position for the specific intervention. For example, indicate patient in sidelying or indicate exercises were provided in a gravity reduced position.
- **Details.** Include the duration, frequency, and number and length of rest breaks.
- **Alterations.** Anything that would not be considered standard practice.
- **Time.** Include the time of each intervention and total treatment time.

In addition, you will want to document the following information related to each of these areas.

Documenting Communication/Coordination

- Any communication with the supervising physical therapist
- Communication with other health care practitioner; for example, physician, registered nurse (RN), occupational therapist (OT), prosthetist
- Conversations with administrators or case managers
- Phone conversations with any of the above

Patient-Related Instruction

- Therapeutic activity instruction; for example, home exercise program (HEP)
- Precautions/restricted activity; for example, total hip precautions or lifting restrictions
- Education related to disease process; for example, what is a stroke?
- Education related to physical therapy procedures; for example, what is ultrasound (US) and why is it used?
- Family/caregiver instruction

Procedural Interventions

Functional Training

- Types
  - Activities of daily living
  - Assistive/adaptive devices
  - Body mechanics
  - Developmental activities
  - Gait and locomotion training
  - Prosthetics and orthotics
  - Wheelchair management skills
- Include in documentation:
  - Specific activity; for example, bed to wheelchair transfers
  - Assistive/adaptive devices used

Infection Control Procedures

- Isolation or sterile techniques used; for example, use of gown and gloves when assisting with therapy exercise

Manual Therapy Techniques

- PROM
  - Side(s) (right or left), joint(s), and motion(s)
  - Number of repetitions or time

- Massage
  - Location
  - Type of massage
  - Amount of time

Physical Agents and Mechanical Agents

- Types
  - Athermal agents
  - Biofeedback
  - Compression therapies
  - Cryotherapy
  - Electrotherapeutic agents
  - Hydrotherapy
  - Superficial and deep thermal agents
  - Traction
- Include in documentation:
  - Physical or mechanical agent used
  - Patient position
  - Specific area treated
  - Exact settings used
  - Duration of treatment

Therapeutic Exercise

- Types
  - Aerobic conditioning
  - Balance and coordination training
  - Conditioning and reconditioning activities
  - Posture awareness training
  - Range of motion exercises
  - Stretching exercises
  - Strengthening exercises
- Include in documentation:
  - Specific activities/exercises performed
  - Equipment used
  - Patient position (if not clear by use of equipment)
  - Repetitions
  - Time spent

Wound Management

- Application and removal of dressings or agents
- Type and amount of dressing used
- Precautions for dressing removal

Equipment Provided

- For example, exercise band for home exercises

Response to All Procedural Interventions

- Can be documented in either O or A (Example 8-1)

TIPS FOR DOCUMENTING RESULTS OF DATA COLLECTED

- When documenting results of data collection, include all information needed for the test to be reproduced and for the results to be clearly understood. Be sure to include the following:
  - Procedure utilized; for example, goniometry, MMT, observation
  - Exactly what was measured; for example, right elbow flexion PROM
  - The patient's position

TYPES OF DATA COLLECTED

Vital Signs (indicate before and/or after exercise/activity as appropriate)

- Heart rate
  - Location
  - Quality
  - Rate
- Respiratory rate
  - Rate
  - Rhythm
  - Depth
  - Regularity of pattern
- Blood pressure
  - Location, side
  - Systolic over diastolic; for example, BP: (R) brachial 120/80

Anthropometric Characteristics

- Height
- Weight
- Length
- Girth

Muscle Strength

- Range; for example, when documenting strength for right elbow flexors document 3/5 instead of 3
- What is measured
  - Muscle group; for example, hip flexors
  - Specific muscles; for example, gluteus maximus
- Arrange logically
  - Group per anatomical location; for example, group shoulder musculature together: shoulder flexors 4/5, extensors 4-/5, abduction 4-/5, adduction 4+/5

- Use tables or columns to show (B) measurement or before/after measurements
- Any deviation from standard position/protocol; for example, tested hip extension in side lying due to pt. unable to get in prone because of obesity

Pain

- Results from written pain questionnaires, scales, and diagrams
  - Examples include the McGill Pain Questionnaire, Pain Disability Index, visual analogue scales, pain drawings, and pain maps
- Note: verbal descriptions of pain given by the patient are written in the subjective portion of the note. Sometimes data from pain questionnaires are also recorded in the subjective portion of the interim note.

Range of Motion

- Document the range from the beginning of the range available to the end of the range available; for example, elbow flexion 5° to 110° instead of just elbow flexion 110°
- Specific joint
- Arrange logically
- Group per anatomical location
- Use tables or columns to show (B) measurements or before/after measurements
- Any deviation from standard position/protocol; for example, shoulder external rotation; unable to achieve standard test position due to pain restrictions; pt. placed in 45° of abduction for measurement

Results of Any Standard Tests or Questionnaires

- Record measurements per the standard of the test being used; for example, Berg Balance Test

DESCRIBING PATIENT FUNCTION

Assistive, Adaptive, Orthotic, Protective, Supportive, and Prosthetic Devices

- Specify device being used; for example, left custom ankle–foot orthosis (AFO).
- Discuss patient's (patient's family's/caregiver's) ability to care for device.
- Discuss patient's ability to don/doff device as appropriate.

- Discuss skin condition related to use of the device.
- Discuss safety risks associated with use of the device.

Gait, Locomotion, and Balance

- Indicate activity; for example, gait or wheelchair mobility.
- Indicate any assistive, adaptive, orthotic, protective, supportive, or prosthetic devices used; for example, wheeled walker.
- Indicate type of surface the patient is traversing; for example, level surface or stairs.
- Indicate distance traveled or amount of time activity is tolerated; for example, 100 feet or 10 minutes.
- List amount and type of physical assistance provided; for example, pt. required min (A) to place (L) LE.
- Number of people needed to provide assistance; for example, pt. required min (A) x 1 indicates 1 person provided minimal assistance. If no number is provide, then assume it is 1 person.
- List amount and type of cues given; for example, pt. required constant verbal cues for cane placement.
- Describe gait pattern used if appropriate; for example, 4-point gait pattern.
- Describe gait deviations if appropriate; for example, pt. demonstrated (L) foot drop during swing phase of gait.
- When documenting gait include weight-bearing status.

Self-Care, Home Management, and Community or Work Reintegration

- Record measurements of physical environments.
- Record any safety concerns or barriers in home, community, and work environments.

Results of Any Standard Tests or Questionnaires

- Record measurements per the standard of the test being used. For example, Functional Independence Measure (FIM) and SF-36.[1]
- The *Guide to Physical Therapist Practice* provides a comprehensive list of assessment tools and references for their associated reliability and validity as reported in the literature.

In order to provide greater objectivity and reliability when documenting functional status, some clinics and facilities utilize standardized tests or questionnaires to measure impairments, function, and degree of disability. Each test or questionnaire will have specific directions related to appropriate documentation to allow for consistency of administration and scoring. When utilizing a standardized tool, the clinician and facility will want to verify its validity and reliability. Specific tools are designed for specific patient populations. A tool that has been determined to be valid in one setting may not be appropriate in another. Finally, traditional grading of function (independent, minimal assistance, etc) should be consistent with scoring given on standardized instruments. Table 8-1 demonstrates a comparison of documentation of functional status utilizing traditional terminology and scoring utilizing a standardized test for measuring a patient's function, the FIM. Other functional measures can be found in Table 8-2 and on the Rehab Measures Database at www.rehabmeasures.org.

OBSERVATIONS

Arousal, Mentation, and Cognition

- Describe changes in patient's state of arousal, mentation, and cognition; for example, pt. lethargic today; difficult to arouse and attend to therapeutic activities

Integumentary Integrity

- Location of wound/skin condition
- Size of wound
- Depth of wound
- Location and depth of any tunneling/undermining
- Description of tissue
- Description of surrounding area
- Description of drainage
- Description of odor
- Activities, positioning, and postures that aggravate or relieve pain, alter sensation, or produce associated skin trauma

Joint Integrity and Mobility

- Describe abnormal joint movements/end feels

Muscle Performance

- Describe abnormal muscle mass; for example, left lower extremity gastrocnemius atrophy compared to right lower extremity
- Describe change in muscle tone; for example, noted hypertonicity of right lower extremity during gait with straight cane

Neuromotor Development

- Describe gross and fine motor milestones
- Describe abnormal righting and equilibrium reactions

Table 8-1

DOCUMENTATION OF FUNCTIONAL STATUS USING TRADITIONAL TERMINOLOGY VERSUS FIM SCORES

Abbrev.	Definition	Amount/Type of Assistance Needed	FIM Score	Descriptor	Amount/Type of Assistance Needed
(I)	Independent	No assistance needed	7	Complete independence	All of the tasks described as making up the activity are typically performed safely, without modification, assistive devices, or aids, and within a reasonable amount of time
No direct correlation with FIM score			6	Modified independence	One or more of the following may be true: • The activity requires an assistive device • The activity takes more than reasonable time • There are safety risks
SBA	Standby assist	Needs someone close by for safety or to provide verbal or visual cues	5	Supervision or setup	Subject requires no more help than standby, cueing or coaxing, without physical contact or helper sets up needed items or applies orthoses or assistive/adaptive devices
CGA	Contact guard assist	Needs someone touching the patient for safety or to provide physical cues	No direct correlation with FIM scores		
Min	Minimal	Pt. performs 75% or more of the effort	4	Minimal contact assistance	Subject requires no more help than touching and expends 75% or more of the effort
Mod	Moderate	Pt. performs 25% to 75% of the effort	3	Moderate assistance	Subject requires more help than touching or expends half or more of the effort (50% to 75%)
Max	Maximal	Pt. performs 25% or less of the activity	2	Maximal assistance	Subject expends less than 50% of the effort but at least 25%

Pain

- Describe patient's nonverbal pain responses to activities, positioning, and postures
- Pain questionnaires

Posture

- Describe alignment of trunk
- Describe alignment of extremities in relation to the trunk

Ventilation, Respiration, and Circulation Examination

- Describe skin color in relation to circulation and ventilation
- Describe symptoms of ventilation/respiratory or circulatory deficiency
- Describe chest wall expansion and excursion
- Describe cough
- Describe sputum color and consistency

Table 8-2

OUTCOME MEASURES AND THEIR TARGET PATIENT POPULATION

Outcome Measure	Patient Population
Acute Care Index of Function (ACIF)	Acute neurological
Arthritis Impact Measurement Scale (AIMS2)	Arthritis
Asthma Quality of Life Questionnaires	Asthma
Cardiac Health Profile	Cardiovascular disease
Dallas Pain Questionnaire	Chronic spinal pain
Diabetes Impact Measurement Scale (DIMS)	Type 1 and Type 2 diabetes
Disability Rating Scale	Severe head trauma
Fatigue Impact Scale	Chronic disease
Fibromyalgia Impact Questionnaire	Fibromyalgia
Foot Function Index	Foot pain
Frail Elderly Functional Assessment	Frail elderly
Functional Independence Measure (FIM)	Variety
Functional Performance Inventory	Moderate to severe COPD
Fugl-Meyer Assessment Scale	CVA
Gross Motor Performance Measure (GMPM)	Children with cerebral palsy
Gross Motor Function Measure (GMFM)	Pediatric
Harris Hip Scale	Hip arthritis
Neck Disability Index (NDI)	Neck disorders
Oswestry Low Back Pain Disability Questionnaire	Low back disorders
Parkinson's Disease Quality of Life (PDQL)	Parkinson's disease
Patient-Rated Wrist Evaluation (PRWE)	Wrist disorders
Peabody Development Motor Scales	Pediatric motor development
Pediatric Evaluation of Disability Index (PEDI)	Pediatric
Physical Disability Index	Frail elderly
SF-12	Variety
SF-36	Variety
Sickness Impact Profile (SIP)	Variety with versions for nursing home residents and stroke
Stroke Impact Scale	CVA
Therapeutic Associates Outcomes System	Variety of musculoskeletal disorders
Western Ontario and McMaster Universities Osteoarthritis Index	Osteoarthritis
WeeFIM	Pediatric function

REFERENCE

1. American Physical Therapy Association. *The Guide to Physical Therapist Practice*. Alexandria, Va: American Physical Therapy Association; 2001. Available at guidetoptpractice.apta.org. Accessed February 18, 2012.

REVIEW QUESTIONS

1. Describe the type(s) of information that should be documented in the objective portion of a SOAP note.

2. Define *reliability* and *validity*.

3. How are data from tests and measures used by the PTA to make decisions about provision of selected interventions? How can limitations of objective data can be minimized and controlled?

4. When is it important for the PTA to document data indicating that body structures and functions or activities are within normal limits?

5. When can tables or columns be used to document objective information? What are the benefits of structuring the information in this format?

APPLICATION EXERCISES

I. Review *The Guide to Physical Therapist Practice* list of categories for tests and measurements. Choose one category from tests and measures (ie, aerobic capacity and endurance) and identify *one* specific test/measure that can be used to collect data for that category. Identify the tools and procedures used for the test. Research the reliability and validity of that test. Indicate whether the test measures an impairment or function (ie, disability, activity limitation, or participation restriction).

II. Write the following statements in a more clear and concise manner, as it would appear in the medical record.
    1. The child walked from the classroom to the cafeteria (~500') with the PTA providing ~25% assistance using Lofstrand crutches. She required cues at the trunk for rotation and upper and lower body dissociation. She used a 4-point gait pattern. Her lower extremities were externally rotated and knees were in a valgus position. Hips were adducted.

    2. The patient was able to walk in the hallway at the hospital with supervision and no assistive device. Her velocity was 0.8m/sec.

    3. The patient demonstrated the following range of motion measurements: passive range of motion for right shoulder flexion was 115° and for shoulder extension 10°.

    4. The patient propelled his wheelchair down the hallway, onto the elevator, and up and down the ramp in the front of the school. The total distance was ~1000 feet. He required 2 rest breaks for ~2 minutes each. He needed minimal assist to ascend the ramp and turn the wheelchair on the elevator.

    5. Prior to initiating interventions the measurements taken for the cardiovascular system were blood pressure at 135 systolic and 90 diastolic, heart rate at 98 beats per minute, the patient's oxygen saturation was 98%, and his respiratory rate was 12 breaths per minute.

III. Organize the following information so that it is clear, concise, and suitable for entry into the medical record.
    1. The patient's AROM is as follows: Right knee flexion 100°, right knee extension 5°, right hip abduction 20°, right hip flexion 100°, right ankle plantarflexion 20°, left elbow 10°–100°, left shoulder flexion 100°, left shoulder abduction 100°, right hip internal rotation 20°, right ankle dorsiflexion 5°, left shoulder external rotation 60°, left shoulder internal rotation 45°, left hip abduction 25°, left hip extension 0°, right hip extension 5°, right elbow flexion 120°, right elbow extension 0°, right shoulder flexion 165°, left knee flexion 120°, left hip flexion 120°, left hip internal rotation 20°, left hip external rotation 40°, right hip external rotation 45°, left knee extension 0°, left plantarflexion 45°, left dorsiflexion 20°, right shoulder abduction 140°, right shoulder external rotation 80°, and right shoulder internal rotation 45°.

2. You are working with an 8-month-old child with hypotonia and developmental delay. She was able to maintain prone on elbows for 2 minutes independently while given a visual cue. She was able to prop sit with supervision for 30 seconds. The infant was also able to demonstrate a righting reaction to the right but not to the left.

3. The patient with cervical radiculopathy had the following neck active range of motion measurements: cervical flexion 30° with pain, extension 20°, right lateral flexion 30°, left lateral flexion 25°. His treatment included moist heat for 15 minutes, soft tissue massage for 10 minutes, 20 repetitions each chin tucks and scapular retractions. He was educated on lifting mechanics and postural correction. He also received intermittent mechanical traction with 15 pounds of pressure with 30 seconds on and 10 seconds off for 10 minutes.

4. The patient with right hemiplegia was able to ambulate 50′ twice with a large-based quad cane. She required minimal assist for guarding at her trunk, but moderate to maximum assist for achieving full swing, placing the right foot, and stabilizing the right knee during midstance.

5. Wound assessment revealed the following information. The skin around the wound is red, warm to the touch, shiny, and swollen. The wound is a 4 cm × 2.4 cm oval-shaped wound on the dorsum of the foot. It is 1.5 cm deep. The patient has diminished sensation to light touch when compared bilateral. She is unable to feel the 10g monofilament on the plantar surface of the right foot. Girth at the right metatarsophalangeal (MTP) joins is 22 cm and 18 cm on the left. The right dorsal pedis pulse is present but diminished compared to the (L), which is 2+.

IV. Review the objective portion of a SOAP note as found in Example 8-2. Critique the note by answering the following questions:
   1. Is the information structured logically?

   2. Is the information presented in a way that allows for ease of finding pertinent information?

   3. Does the objective information provide data that addresses impairment and function?

   4. Does the objective information provide data about the patient's activity limitations or participation restrictions?

   5. Does the objective information provide data about the patient's overall disabilities?

V. While working with a patient in a skilled nursing facility who is recovering from a left total hip arthroplasty, the following information is obtained. Organize and write the information so that it is clear, concise, and suitable for entry as an interim note.

   Prior to initiating interventions the following data were gathered: The blood pressure reading was 130/85, heart rate was 88 beats per minute and respiratory rate was 20 breaths per minute. There was a scar that appeared to be healing well on the left hip, surgical staples were present and intact, and there was no drainage from the wound. The following data were gathered during or after the interventions: The patient's left knee musculature measured at a 4+ out of 5 and the ankle musculature measured 5 out of 5. The assistant helped the patient walk in the hallway. The patient was able to walk 50 feet while the assistant provided about 25% assistance. The patient used a standard walker. The assistant provided verbal instructions for sequencing and encouragement to put as much weight as the patient felt comfortable with through the leg. The patient also occasionally placed the walker too far in front of her and the

Example 8-2

Objective: (L) Knee ROM: Active   Passive
                           0° to 125°   0° to 135°

Hamstring Length: In supine lacks 50° knee extension with hip at 90° flexion

Gastrocnemius Length: In supine with knee fully extended DF PROM was 0° to 5°

Strength: (L) quadriceps 3−/5; (L) hamstrings 3/5; patient has marked pain with resisted knee extension. Pain is most keenly felt over the mid portion of the patellar tendon.

Gait: Ambulates with one axillary crutch in the (R) hand and knee immobilizer in place. Gait noted after removal of the immobilizer, the patient keeps the affected knee in strict extension.

therapist had to remind the patient of the proper walker placement. When the assistant helped the patient up from the bed the patient needed 25% assistance to scoot over in bed. The assistant primarily helped by moving the operative limb. When sitting upon the side of the bed the patient required more assistance and was able to perform about 50% of the activity. When moving from sitting on the edge of the bed to standing with the walker the patient performed about 50% of the task.

Chapter 9

Writing the Assessment and Plan

Rebecca McKnight, PT, MS

CHAPTER OBJECTIVES

After reading this chapter, the student will be able to do the following:

1. List the type of information that should be recorded in the assessment portion of a SOAP note.
2. List the type of information that should be recorded in the plan portion of a SOAP note.
3. Describe the importance of the assessment and plan portions of a note in relationship to reimbursement.
4. Organize given information into a logically structured and well-written assessment portion of a SOAP note.
5. Organize given information into a logically structured and well-written plan portion of a SOAP note.
6. Describe the importance of linking assessment and plan information in the interim note with information in the evaluative note.
7. Organize given information into a complete, logically structured SOAP note following basic documentation guidelines.

INTRODUCTION

The assessment section of the interim SOAP note answers the question, "What does it all mean?" This is the PT's or PTA's opportunity to explain the relevance of the documented data. The assessment is often the most difficult section of the note to write but is definitely the most important. A key point to remember about writing the assessment to is to provide a picture of why skilled services are needed. This is the PT's or PTA's (where allowed by law) opportunity to summarize the patient's progress (or lack thereof), status toward goals, changes in condition, ongoing impairments, activity limitations, and participation restrictions. This is the place to make obvious how interventions have led to changes in the patient's status. Imagine that you are talking with an insurance company, and you really want to portray the patient's status.

The assessment section provides a summary of the S and O information. In this section you should also include an explanation of how the data demonstrate the patient's response to the intervention(s) provided and a statement about how the patient is progressing in reference to the goals established in the initial plan of care.

IMPORTANCE OF DOCUMENTING THE ASSESSMENT (A)

As stated in Chapter 2, appropriate documentation is required in order to meet ethical and legal standards and to communicate with reimbursement bodies like Medicare and Medicaid. It is within the assessment section of the SOAP note that the PT and PTA are able to document the patient's need for physical therapy services by showing how the recommended plan of care requires the skills of a PT or PTA.

When applicable, you should indicate how interventions have led to the changes in the patient's status. Information in the assessment section should clearly describe the patient's response to the intervention(s) provided and the patient's progress in reference to the goals established in the plan of care. This information should clearly demonstrate

Erickson M, McKnight R. *Documentation Basics:*
A Guide for the Physical Therapist Assistant, Second Edition (pp. 91-96)
© 2012 SLACK Incorporated

why continuation of skilled services is needed. You will need to be concise but also specific. General phrases like, "The patient tolerated the treatment well" or "The patient is progressing toward stated goals" should be avoided.[1]

EXPLANATION OF HOW THE DATA DEMONSTRATE THE PATIENT'S RESPONSE TO INTERVENTION

- **Change in pain level**. For example, you are providing TENS application for pain control for a patient with chronic back pain with radicular symptoms. Prior to initiating intervention, the patient rates his pain as 7/10. The patient rates his pain as 2/10 after initiation of TENS trial.
- **Change in impairment**. For example, you are assisting with the care of a patient who has lymphedema. You are using volumetric measurements to document the amount of edema before and after intervention.
- **Change in functional status**. For example, you are working in an outpatient clinic with a 32-year-old male who injured his back playing football with friends. When he enters the clinic, his complaints of pain and stiffness caused him to be unable to bend over to take off his shoes. After receiving physical agents and appropriate therapeutic exercise, the patient is able to put on his shoes to leave the clinic.

PATIENT'S PROGRESS TOWARD GOALS

Indicate the following:
- Whether a goal has been achieved
- Progress toward a goal
- No progress toward a goal
- A decline in patient status (Example 9-1)

Tips

- There should never be any information in the assessment section that does not relate to data documented in S and O sections.
- Back up all statements with data from the S and O sections. For example, if you document that the patient has an improvement in his or her mobility, refer to the data documented in the O section that substantiates that comment.
- Be specific. Do not document "Tolerated treatment well" or "Patient progressing." Always indicate how you know these things.[1]
- In keeping with the ICF disablement model,[2] you should indicate relationships between impairments, activity limitations, and participation restrictions in this section. For example, the following statement

---

Example 9-1

A: Showing improvement in ROM and strength and functional gait. Pt. has met STGs 2 & 3. Will cont. to work toward STGs 1&4 and all LTGs.

---

would be very appropriate: A: Patient continues to have decreased AROM in the (R) shoulder limiting her ability to dress and reach into her overhead cabinets.
- The effect of the interventions on activity limitations and participation restrictions should be highlighted. For example, A: Pt. demonstrating improved ROM in the (R) shoulder since starting HEP. Improvement in ROM has allowed better ability to dress and reach into overhead cabinets.

PLAN (P)

The final component of a SOAP note is the plan. The plan section of an interim SOAP note answers the question, "Where do we go from here?" The plan should be based on the established plan of care and the patient's response to the interventions and progression toward goals. The plan will delineate what actions need to occur within the 3 areas of intervention: (1) coordination/communication and documentation, (2) patient/client-related instructions, and (3) procedural interventions. Types of information that can be included in the plan section of an interim note include the following:
- Coordination/communication and documentation
  - Request for a re-examination/re-evaluation by the PT; for example, the patient is not progressing as desired with the current plan of care/treatment plan.
  - Communication with other health care providers; for example, discussing discharge plans with a social worker.
- Patient/client-related instructions
  - Written instruction to be provided; for example, will issue and instruct in home exercise program (HEP) next session.
  - Education regarding activity restrictions and precautions; for example, will educate patient regarding hip precautions and car transfers.
- Procedural interventions
  - Progression of treatment plan within established plan of care; for example, will increase resistance with therapeutic exercises.
  - Modification of treatment plan within established plan of care; for example, will change from using a standard walker to using a wheeled walker due to the patient's continued problems with appropriate sequencing while using the standard walker.

Example 9-2

P: Cont PT in the outpatient setting 3x/wk for strengthening, ROM, and proprioceptive exercises and gait training.

Jody Laughlin, PTA

○ Equipment to be purchased; for example, wheeled walker for home use.

○ Activities to perform; for example, will focus on bed mobility training.

○ Schedule for continued therapy; for example, to continue with twice daily treatments with anticipated discharge in 3 days to home.

Tips

- Use phrases such as "Will check," "Will update," "Will consult," "Will increase," "Will hold."
- The plan should include anything that you are thinking about doing with the patient.
- Indicate why treatments you are planning are medically necessary; for example, will initiate light strengthening next visit to reduce atrophy and weakness associated with immobilization.
- This should serve as a reminder to you during the patient's next session and provide a guide for the next therapist or assistant treating the patient (Example 9-2).

Now that you know basic documentation principles and specific guidelines for documenting patient care in a SOAP note format, you should be able to adapt and document this information in an appropriate manner regardless of the policies and styles you are presented with in the clinical situations you encounter.

PULLING IT ALL TOGETHER

The APTA's *Guidelines for Physical Therapy Documentation* indicate that "documentation is required for every patient visit/encounter."[3] The primary purposes of a treatment, interim, or daily note is to document what occurred during that session or on that day in relation to the patient's physical therapy services and to support the billing codes that were used. Documentation of the patient visit should include the following elements: (1) subjective reports from the patient, (2) specific interventions provided during the session that are consistent with what was billed, (3) any equipment or written instruction provided to the patient,

(4) the patient's response to the interventions provided including objective improvements made, (5) any factor leading to a modification of the plan of care, and (6) any communication or collaboration with other health providers regarding the patient's care.[3] To ease time constraints and facilitate consistency between clinicians, interventions are often documented through the use of standard forms, checklists, flowsheets, or graphs.

STRUCTURE OF AN INTERIM SOAP NOTE

The structure and organization of a SOAP interim note will be similar to the structure and organization of the examination/evaluation note. At the beginning of the note you will need to provide the patient's name and the date the services were provided. The subjective section includes patient remarks regarding his or her condition, the intervention, and changes in impairment or function brought on by the treatment. When documenting objective data, it is important to clearly differentiate between tests and measurement data that have been collected to illustrate the patient's status and interventions that were provided. The latter is frequently accomplished by the utilization of tables or flowsheets for documentation of specific interventions. Alternatively, this can be accomplished by using subheadings (ie, *Impairments, Functional Status, Coordination of Care, Patient-Related Instruction,* and *Procedural Interventions*). As noted earlier in this chapter, the assessment section should include information regarding the patient's response to the interventions provided as well as progress toward stated goals. It is important to reference both the initial evaluation and the information found in the subjective and objective sections of the interim note to craft the assessment information. The note ends with the PTA outlining what activities will occur in the future related to the patient's physical therapy care. Finally, you will need to sign your name.

REFERENCES

1. Clifton DW Jr. "Tolerated treatment well" may no longer be tolerated. *PT Magazine.* 1995;3(10):24.
2. World Health Organization. *The International Classification of Functioning, Disability, and Health.* Last Updated: 2001. http://whqlibdoc.who.int/publications/2001/9241545429.pdf. Accessed February 24, 2011.
3. American Physical Therapy Association. *The Guide to Physical Therapist Practice.* Alexandria, Va: American Physical Therapy Association; 2001. Available at guidetoptpractice.apta.org. Accessed February 18, 2012.

REVIEW QUESTIONS

1. What type of information is found within the assessment and plan portions of the SOAP note?

2. How should an interim note be structured? How should the information relate to the initial evaluation?

APPLICATION EXERCISES

I. Write the following information in a clear, concise manner, as it would appear in the medical record.

1. Upon arrival in the outpatient department for her follow-up visit, the patient indicated that she has been doing her HEP without any problems and that she feels that she is able to don her coat, reach for her car door and seat belt, and perform light household chores without difficulty.

2. You have been treating a patient with plantar fasciitis, providing ultrasound, soft tissue massage, and stretching. On the third visit, the patient indicates his pain in the morning has decreased from 5/10 to 3/10. His active and passive dorsiflexion range of motion have increased 5°. During gait, he has increased his stance time on the involved extremity.

3. The 8-year-old child with spastic diplegia is now able to walk with standby assist from her classroom to the bathroom (~150') with a posterior walker. At the beginning of the school year (3 months ago), she was only able to walk 50' with minimal assist of 1.

4. You are assisting an 18-year-old female who injured her knee playing basketball in walking with crutches. The patient walks in the hallway for 100' without your help. When the patient attempts to walk up the stairs, she tells you it scares her. You have to keep a hand on her to provide minimal stability for her to get up and down one flight of stairs. At the last visit, she could only ascend and descend 3 steps. You are planning to continue with increasing her independence on the stairs. She is not allowed to bear any weight on the injured lower extremity.

5. You are working with a 42-year-old patient recovering from spinal meningitis. The patient currently needs moderate assistance to perform transfers to and from the wheelchair with a slideboard. The patient also requires occasional verbal cues for setting up the equipment for the transfer. Last week, the patient required maximum assist for the slideboard transfer. The initial plan of care includes a goal for the patient to be independent. You plan on continuing with slideboard transfers and mobility training bid.

II. The following is an initial examination and evaluation for a patient recently admitted to an inpatient rehab hospital. Use it to help you complete the following 2 SOAP notes.

Initial Examination and Evaluation

Pr: (L) CVA, (R) hemiparesis

Hx: This 67-y.o. male was admitted to the acute care 08-08-11 due to sudden weakness in his (R) UE & LE and slurred speech. Pt.'s PMH includes NIDDM, CABG x 2 07-05-08. No other pertinent medical history.

S: *c/o:* Inability to move around like he used to. Weakness in (R) LE & UE. *Prior level of function:* (I) c̄ all ADLs and gait s̄ assistive device. Active; worked in his woodshop, yard, and garden. Pt. is (R) handed. *Home situation:* Lives c̄ wife who is healthy but is a small woman. Lives in 2-level home c̄ 4 steps to enter.

O: *Observation:* Noted 3+ pitting edema in (R) hand and forearm; pt. has tendency to keep (R) UE in dependent position.
Sensation: Pt. displays diminished light touch, deep pressure localization, proprioception & kinesthesia through the (R) UE & LE.
Tone: Pt. displays diminished tone on (R) UE & LE to passive range, diminished patellar reflexes and absent Achilles reflex on (R).
MMT: (L) UE & LE: 5/5 throughout all musculature. (R) UE: shoulder flex, ext, abd, MR&LR 2–/5; elbow flex 2+/5, ext 2/5; grip 1/5; (R) LE: hip ext, add, IR 3+/5; flex, add, LR 2+/5; knee ext 3–/5, flex 2–/5; ankle DF 0/5, PF 1/5.
Mobility: Max (A) scooting up in bed, mod (A) scooting (R) & (L) in bed; SBA for safety and v/c when rolling to (R); max (A) rolling to (L).
Transfers: Supine ↔ sit max (A) x 1 from (R) side and mod (A) x 1 from (L) side; sit to stand max (A) x 1; stand pivot w/c ↔ bed max (A) x 1.
Gait: Not attempted at this time.
Balance: Fair– static and poor dynamic sitting balance; standing balance very poor.
Endurance: Fair; pt. tolerated 30-minute session requiring 1-minute rest breaks every 5–8 minutes.

A: PT Dx: Impaired motor function and muscular performance due to CVA. Prognosis is good for goals as stated. Skilled service needed to help patient improve strength and functional mobility including gait and transfers so that he can return home.
Problem List:
- Edema in (R) UE
- Decreased strength (R) UE & LE
- Dependent bed mobility
- Dependent transfers
- Nonambulatory
- Diminished balance
- Diminished endurance

STGs to be met in 2 weeks:
1. Pt. will be able to demonstrate understanding of appropriate positioning for (R) UE.
2. Pt. will demonstrate an increase in strength (R) UE & LE ½ grade throughout to allow improved mobility and use of UE.
3. Pt. will require mod (A) scooting up in bed, min (A) scooting (R) & (L) in bed; mod (A) rolling to (L) and be (I) rolling to (R).
4. Pt. will require mod (A) for supine to sit from (R), min (A) supine to sit from (L), mod (A) for sit ↔ stand and w/c ↔ bed transfers.
5. Pt. will stand c̄ max (A) x 1 and quad cane for 1 minute.
6. Pt. will display fair static and fair– dynamic sitting balance and fair– static standing balance.
7. Pt. will display adequate endurance to tolerate a 30-minute therapy session only needing one 2-minute rest break.

LTGs to be met in 4 weeks:
1. Pt. will be (I) in (R) UE self-care.
2. Pt. will demonstrate an increase in strength (R) UE & LE 1 grade throughout to allow improved mobility and use of UE.
3. Pt. will be (I) c̄ bed mobility including scooting up and down in bed and rolling to (R) or (L).
4. Pt. will be (I) c̄ sit ↔ stand and w/c ↔ bed transfers.
5. Pt. will ambulate 20' c̄ assistive device as indicated and mod (A) x 1 to allow some household ambulation.

6. Pt. will display good static and dynamic sitting balance, fair+ static and fair dynamic standing balance.
7. Pt. will display adequate endurance for a one hour session of therapy c̄ only one 5-minute rest break.

P: PT bid for neuromuscular re-education, strengthening, mobility training, pre-gait activities, endurance activities, balance training, and education related to positioning and self-care.

Mary Jane, DPT

1.   Today the patient states that he feels he is getting stronger and is looking forward to his first day pass to go home with his wife this weekend. The patient's wife states that she is concerned about how they will manage in the long run. She says that their son and daughter-in-law are coming in from out of town to help out this weekend. In therapy today you worked on his bed mobility and transfers. He needed moderate assistance when scooting up and down in bed and scooting to the right. He needed minimal assistance when scooting to the left. He was able to roll to the right without any assistance and was safe with the activity. He required moderate assistance when rolling to the left. The patient still displays significant edema in his right hand and forearm and forgets to use his positioning devices in bed and in the wheelchair. He required minimal assistance when coming up from his left side. He required minimal assistance when performing a sit-to-stand transfer and moderate assistance with a stand pivot transfer from the therapy mat into the wheelchair. You educated the patient's wife regarding his need for supervision and constant verbal cues to perform wheelchair setup and because he is impulsive and unsafe at times. Review the initial evaluative note so that you can make appropriate comparisons with his initial status. Be sure to include a summary of how he is progressing toward his goals and write an appropriate plan.

2.   One week later, the patient has returned from a weekend pass with his family. The family had considerable difficulty caring for the patient at home and they feel the home is not set up well for caring for him. The patient is upset at how difficult it was to be at home. He needs a lot of extra encouragement today to participate in therapy. During his therapy session today the patient required moderate to maximal assistance with rolling and scooting in bed and for supine to sit transfers when coming up from his right side, and minimal assistance when coming up from his left side. He required maximal assistance when performing a sit-to-stand transfer and moderate assistance with a modified stand pivot transfer from the therapy mat into the wheelchair. The patient needed moderate assistance and constant verbal cues to perform setup and was impulsive and a safety risk today more than usual due to his bad mood associated with his weekend. In your note, include a summary of how these findings compare with findings from the previous note and the initial evaluative note. Also briefly comment on the status of his goals and write an appropriate plan.

Chapter 10

Payment Basics

Mia L. Erickson, PT, EdD, CHT, ATC

Chapter Objectives

After reading this chapter, the student will be able to do the following:

1. Define *reimbursement*.
2. Differentiate between first-, second-, and third-party payers.
3. Differentiate between different types of insurance (social, managed care, casualty, and indemnity).
4. Explain the difference between Medicare Parts A, B, C, and D and Medicaid.
5. Examine Medicare reimbursement in a variety of settings (inpatient hospitals, inpatient rehabilitation hospitals, skilled nursing facilities, home health care, and outpatient facilities).
6. Examine strategies for cost containment utilized by managed care organizations.
7. Define *pro bono*.
8. Construct a physical therapy progress note using basic principles for maximum reimbursement.
9. Realize how documentation is tied to reimbursement.

What Is Reimbursement?

There are generally 3 parties involved in the financial management of an individual's medical care: (1) the patient (first party); (2) the health care provider, such as the physician, physical therapist, occupational therapist, etc (second party); and (3) the insurance company (third party). When a patient receives a service from a health care provider, some form of payment is expected. This payment can

come directly from the patient (first-party payment), but more often it comes from the patient's insurance company. Payment to the health care provider from the insurance company is known as third-party payment or reimbursement. The APTA has defined *reimbursement* as payment by the patient (first-party) or insurer (third-party) to the health care provider for services provided.[1] Third-party payment accounts for more than 80% of all payments for rehabilitative care.[2] The financial success and viability of physical therapy departments and clinics is dependent upon payment from patients or third-party payers. In the past, physical therapists were paid, or reimbursed, 100% of what they billed. Today, however, this is not the case. Instead, providers are usually paid a percentage of what is billed. There are also many rules and regulations governing the amount of money paid to providers for their services, and they vary according to different insurance companies, insurance policies and contracts, and payers.

Types of Payment

As you begin your clinical affiliations and begin to practice as a PTA, you will realize that physical therapists receive different types of payment. A brief description of common payment structures is provided in this chapter. For more detail, the APTA's Web site is a valuable resource for reimbursement questions.

Social Insurance

Social insurance is a type of insurance where money is directed from individuals who can pay to those who cannot. Examples are Medicare, Medicaid, and state programs for

97

Erickson M, McKnight R. *Documentation Basics: A Guide for the Physical Therapist Assistant, Second Edition (pp. 97-104)*
© 2012 SLACK Incorporated

individuals who do not have health insurance.[2] The Social Security Act of 1965 established Medicare and Medicaid to provide the elderly and the poor with health insurance coverage.[3] In 1972, Medicare benefits were extended to individuals with disabilities and those with permanent kidney failure.[3] Today, Medicare provides benefits to the following[4]:

- People 65 years of age and older
- People younger than 65 with certain disabilities
- Individuals with end-stage renal disease (ESRD; ie, permanent kidney failure with dialysis or transplant).

From 1977 to 2001, Medicare and Medicaid services were coordinated under the Health Care Financing Administration (HCFA). In 2001, HCFA changed its name to the Centers for Medicare & Medicaid Services (CMS).[5] CMS is a federal agency housed in the Department of Health and Human Services. CMS administers the Medicare program and oversees individual state Medicaid programs.[6] CMS also administers the Children's Health Insurance Program (CHIP) program, a program for uninsured children.[7]

Medicare

The original Medicare program is a federally funded program that consists primarily of 2 parts—Medicare Part A and Medicare Part B. Medicare Part A, or Hospital Insurance Part A, pays for inpatient hospital stays, skilled nursing facilities (SNFs), hospice, and some home health care.[8] It does not cover long-term care or nursing homes. Medicare beneficiaries (individuals who receive Medicare benefits) typically do not pay a fee for Medicare Part A. This payment came from monthly payroll deductions while the individual was employed. Also, enrollment in Part A is automatic for individuals receiving Social Security benefits. Medicare Part B, or Medical Insurance Part B, pays for physician services, outpatient services, durable medical equipment (DME) like walkers and hospital beds, some preventative services, and some services not covered under Part A, like physical and occupational therapy. Enrollment in Medicare Part B is optional. In order to receive benefits under Part B, individuals are required to enroll and pay a monthly premium (~$116.00 per month in 2011 or more dependent on income). This amount is deducted from their monthly Social Security benefit payment and can vary on a year-to-year basis.

Other parts of Medicare include Parts C and D. Medicare Part C consists of Medicare Advantage Plans. These plans are offered and administered by private insurance companies that are approved by Medicare. Part C includes both Part A and Part B (and in some instances Part D) as described above, but each of the advantage plans has different costs and coverage.[8] Beneficiaries may choose to enroll in original Medicare or Part C. Part C has additional costs in addition to the Part B costs. Medicare Part D is Medicare's Prescription Drug Coverage and is optional for Medicare beneficiaries.

For original Medicare Parts A and B, home health care, and DME coverage, Medicare contracts with private insurance companies to pay the bills. For Part A and some Part B, these companies are known as *fiscal intermediaries* (FIs) or *intermediaries*. For Part B, they are known as *carriers*.[9] Regional home health intermediaries (RHHIs) pay bills for home health care and monitor its quality, and durable medical equipment regional carriers (DMERCs) pay bills for durable medical equipment. These fiscal intermediaries and carriers are determined based on geographic regions. It is important to know the payers for your region so that you can become familiar with their reimbursement and documentation guidelines, as they may differ.

Medicare reimbursement varies depending on the type of facility in which you practice. Different payment systems are in place for different practice settings. *Prospective payment systems* (PPS) are a type of Medicare reimbursement based on a predetermined, fixed amount.[10] A PPS is in place for acute care hospitals, inpatient rehabilitation hospitals, skilled nursing facilities, long-term care hospitals, home health care, hospice, hospital outpatient departments, and inpatient psychiatric facilities.[10] Under PPS, the payment amount is derived from patient classification systems specific to the setting (acute care, rehabilitation, skilled nursing facility, etc). Upon admission to one these facilities or services, patients are "grouped" according to common characteristics such as diagnosis, disease, needs and/or functional status. These are known as *case-mix groups*.[11] For each case-mix group, Medicare has agreed to reimburse a predetermined fixed amount. The facility's admissions data or, in some settings, data from standardized evaluation tools, are used to assign patients to a case-mix group.

The PPS in inpatient acute care hospitals is known as *inpatient PPS*, or IPPS. Under the IPPS, each patient is categorized into a diagnosis-related group (DRG). A DRG is a classification system used to group patients according to diagnosis, type of treatment, age, and other relevant criteria.[11] Hospitals are paid a set, predetermined amount according to the patient's DRG category, regardless of the actual cost to provide care to the patient.[11]

Reimbursement provided to SNFs can occur through Part A or Part B. Payment under Part A is determined through information provided about each patient upon his or her admission. This is known as a *case-mix classification system*.[12] For each patient entering an SNF, a minimum data set (MDS) assessment is completed.[13] This is a multidisciplinary assessment performed by a variety of health care providers (physician, physical therapist, occupational therapist, speech therapist, nurse, etc) that includes data such as ADL status, hearing, speech, vision, functional status, and cognitive patterns.[13] Data from the MDS are then used to determine the patient's resource utilization group (RUG) classification. The RUG classification is a hierarchy for grouping patients according to the amount of resources they will need during their stay at an SNF.[13] For example, more complex patients require more staff resources; therefore, facilities are reimbursed at a higher rate.

Reimbursement to inpatient rehabilitation facilities (IRFs) is similar to that for an SNF, with a few exceptions. Like SNFs, upon admission to an IRF, patients are assessed using an inpatient rehabilitation facility patient assessment instrument (IRF PAI). These data are used to classify patients based on clinical characteristics and anticipated resource needs.[14] Payments are determined based on the patient's classification. However, the Functional Independence Measure (FIM) is the integral part of the IRF PAI for rehabilitation practitioners in these settings.[15] The FIM is administered on all patients in this setting, and the scores are used as data on the IRF PAI.

Patient case-mix groups in home health care are also determined by assessing data collected during the admissions process, similar to SNFs and IRFs. However, in home health, the assessment tool is known as the Outcome and Assessment Information Set (OASIS).[16] Data from the OASIS are used to categorize patients into 1 of 80 home health resource groups (HHRG), and payment is predetermined for each group. Though the OASIS is not meant to serve as a comprehensive assessment tool, it does require information on additional patient attributes such as sociodemographic, environmental, support system, and health and functional status.[16] The OASIS is also used for home health agency quality improvement and tracking patient outcomes.

As you can see, each setting has unique assessment tools, categories, and guidelines for reimbursement by Medicare. It is important to point out that though reimbursement has been predetermined for each of the case-mix groups, payments can be adjusted based on geographic location and cost of providing services to particularly complex patients. Reimbursement can also be adjusted for teaching hospitals and to providers who treat a large number of patients without insurance. This is known as *case-mix adjustment*.[16] It is important to remember that in the aforementioned settings, the PT evaluation provides information into the multidisciplinary assessment that establishes the amount facilities are reimbursed for a particular patient. It is important for the PT to accurately document all comorbidities, complexities, and functional problems so the patient is accurately categorized.

Reimbursement provided to hospital-based physical therapy outpatient clinics and physical therapy private practices is based on the Medicare physician fee schedule (MPFS).[17] The MPFS is the PPS for physical, occupational, and speech therapy provided in these settings. Fee schedules are predetermined lists of payment amounts for various services or procedures performed by physicians or health care providers.[11] This predetermined amount is also known as the "Medicare allowable." For example, according to the APTA Web site, the Medicare allowable for a physical therapy evaluation is ~$70.00. It is important to point out that in outpatient settings, Medicare will reimburse 80% of the Medicare allowable. The remaining 20% is the patient's responsibility. The remaining 20% is often paid by the patient's secondary insurance, except in cases where the patient does not have secondary insurance. Then the remaining 20% must be paid by the patient. The APTA provides a link to an up-to-date Medicare fee schedule to its members on its Web site.

The Medicare allowable is determined through the use of an elaborate coding system. First, all health care procedures are assigned a code under the current procedural terminology (CPT) coding system.[18] This is a 5-digit code known as the procedure's CPT code. Under the CPT system, physical therapy procedures generally begin with 97.

Each of the CPT codes is then assigned a weight based on (1) provider work value to administer the procedure; (2) the practice expense, or how much it costs to perform a procedure; and (3) the professional liability (malpractice) value.[2] The professional liability value can be thought of as the associated risk involved with administering a procedure. For example, a joint mobilization has a higher weight than application of a hot pack or cold pack because a joint mobilization requires more technical skill and has higher associated risk. The scale used for weighting the procedures is known as the Resource-Based Relative Value Scale (RBRVS).[19] Each CPT code corresponds with an RBRVS value. Once the RBRVS value has been determined, it is multiplied by a conversion factor ($33.9764 in 2011) to establish the Medicare allowable.[20]

Hypothetical example:

Physical therapy evaluation (CPT code 97001)

RBR Value × Conversion Factor = Medicare Allowable

1.99 × $37.3374 = $74.30

After the conversion factor is applied, the dollar value is then adjusted for the geographic region, or practice location, and that becomes the Medicare allowable for the procedure.[2] In addition to Medicare, other third-party payers use the CPT coding system and the RBRVS to establish fee schedules. Nevertheless, the amount reimbursed by Medicare might vary (higher or lower) from the amount reimbursed by private, nongovernment insurance companies. CPT codes and Relative Values can be found on the American Medical Association Web site.[21]

Medicaid

Medicaid is a joint federally and state-funded program that pays for medical care for individuals and families with low incomes, inadequate medical insurance, or no medical insurance.[22] The federal government oversees general guidelines for Medicaid, but specific requirements to enroll are established by individual states.[22] Some groups often eligible include pregnant women with a low income, children with a low family income, and individuals who are blind or disabled. Children 18 and younger might also be eligible for Medicaid benefits if certain criteria are met.

Reimbursement provided by Medicaid is different from Medicare and varies from state to state. You should become aware of Medicaid reimbursement guidelines in your state.

For both Medicare and Medicaid, there are some procedures that are not covered or may not be covered. If a health care provider believes that a patient would benefit from a procedure that may or may not be covered and the patient agrees to pay for it, the provider must have the patient sign an advance beneficiary notice (ABN). An ABN must be signed on each day the service is provided. An ABN serves to provide and verify communication to Medicare and Medicaid beneficiaries of their financial responsibility for services that will be or could be denied. Downloadable copies of an ABN are available on Medicare's Web site.[23]

Managed Care

Managed care is a type of health care in which the insurance company (payer) contracts with health care providers, including physical therapists, to provide services at a reduced cost to its members. These health care providers make up the plan's network.[24] There are different types of managed care plans, including health maintenance organizations (HMOs) and preferred provider organization (PPOs). An HMO only pays for care within their network.[24] A PPO also includes a network of providers but, unlike HMOs, PPOs often include out-of-network coverage, although there is usually an increased cost to the patient (usually around 30% to 40% of the expenses).

In the past, physical therapy providers could submit a bill and expect to be reimbursed 100% of the amount billed. However, that is not the case today. Managed care insurance contracts are negotiated and providers often agree to accept a lower amount in order to be a provider for the particular insurance company or included in the network. Thus, health care providers accept a reduction in the amount or percentage they are reimbursed. In these plans, there is a predetermined fee schedule like the Medicare physician fee schedule.

Managed care organizations as well as many third-party payers use additional strategies to control money paid to providers in order to contain costs. Any of the following may be used:

- Use of a primary care physician to control access to specialist care—At one time, a patient could choose any provider for his or her health care needs. Now, in some managed care plans, the patient's family doctor, or primary care physician (PCP), is the point of access into the health care system. The PCP can then direct the patient's care or refer the patient to a specialist. Under this system, when patients are referred to a specialist through their PCPs, they are provided maximum insurance coverage. However, if they enter the health care system through a non-PCP, their amount of coverage is reduced. PCPs can be general medicine, family medicine, or internal medicine practitioners. They can also be pediatricians or, in some cases, gynecologists/obstetricians.[2]

- Use of a fee schedule—As indicated previously, in the past, a health care provider could expect to be reimbursed 100% of the amount billed. Now insurance companies set limits on how much they will pay providers by implementing a fee-for-service plan, or a fee schedule, similar to the one described for Medicare.

- Requiring prior authorization—When prior authorization is required, the provider must contact the insurance company (payer) prior to providing a service and outline the treatment/services he or she wishes to carry out. The insurance company may or may not give the provider authorization to perform the recommended service. When prior authorization is required, the insurance company does not reimburse services that have not been approved. Payment for orthotics, splints, braces, and/or medical equipment used by PTs and PTAs often requires prior authorization.

- Limiting the number and duration of services provided—Some insurance companies have policies where there is an established limit on the number of physical therapy visits that will be reimbursed. In addition, there might be language stating that services must be provided within a given time frame.[25] Depending on the insurance, there is a large range and a variety of stipulations. For example, a patient might be allowed 6 visits per diagnosis or 25 visits per calendar year, regardless of diagnosis. There are also cases where the patient is allowed 60 visits in a lifetime. Finally, other plans might allow an initial visit(s) and then require prior authorization from the insurer when additional visits are necessary.[25] You should become familiar with guidelines of frequently encountered insurance companies in your setting.

- Requiring a utilization review process—Utilization review is process where an insurance company employee, such as a nurse or case manager, or an external review organization reviews patient cases for medical necessity, appropriateness, and quality of care provided to patients by a health care provider.[1]

- Requiring case management—Case managers direct patients to the most appropriate amount, duration, and type of health services and monitor medical outcomes. Insurance companies may employ case managers or contract with an independent case management agency.

- Use of deductibles and copayments—Many insurance policies include deductibles and copays. These are payments provided to the health care providers that are the patient's responsibility and are part of the insurance coverage plan purchased by the patient. A typical deductible is ~$1000 per year. This means that the patient pays the first $1000 of his or her health care costs and then the remainder is covered by the insurance company. Patients seen for physical therapy following surgery or a hospitalization usually meet their deductible with the surgery or hospital bills. A copayment (or copay) is a dollar amount paid by the patient each time a service is provided. For example, for therapy visits, a patient might be required to pay a $25 copayment per visit. Copayments and deductibles are becoming increasingly higher and more common among third-party payers, shifting more financial responsibility to the patient.

Casualty Insurance

Casualty insurance, such as workers' compensation and auto accident insurance, is insurance for individuals who are injured on the job or in a motor vehicle accident.[2] These claims are usually handled by payers other than health insurance companies. Workers' compensation plans are run by state governments, and reimbursement and benefits vary from state to state. You should become familiar with your state's workers' compensation guidelines for physical therapy reimbursement.

Indemnity Insurance

Indemnity insurance reimburses the patient for their out-of-pocket medical expenses that are covered under the insurance policy. In other words, the patient pays the provider out of pocket and submits a claim to his or her insurance company. The insurance company then reimburses the patient. In the case of indemnity insurance, the insurer does not provide payment to the health care provider; instead, the contract is between the patient and the insurance company.[2]

Cash-Based Services

In first-party payment, or cash-based services, the patient pays the bill in full on each day that services are provided. There are more PT clinics today than ever before incorporating cash-based services along with third-party reimbursement or operating totally through cash-based services. Cash-based services decrease dependence on third-party payers; place additional responsibility on the patient, including his or her role in the care; and eliminate stipulations on the type, amount, frequency, or duration of services.[26] In addition, cash-based services provide daily cash flow into the clinic. The disadvantage is that patients may not be able to afford physical therapy services and, in these cases, educating the patient on the value of physical therapy is critical.[26]

Pro Bono Services

Pro bono is a term that means "for public good." It is a service provided by a professional at no charge. Pro bono services can be provided by PTs and PTAs for patients without insurance, for patients who have no or inadequate coverage for rehabilitation services, or for those who have exhausted their benefits and cannot afford cash-based services. Facilities that provide pro bono services often have their own eligibility requirements, either formal or informal, for determining whether a patient qualifies for pro bono services and for administering those services. A PT might decide to offer a pro bono clinic once a month. Faculty at PT schools sometimes will run a pro bono faculty practice as a service to the community. Regardless of the process for administering pro bono services, documentation requirements still apply and the episode of care must be documented as if the patient were receiving insurance benefits. In addition, determining to whom pro bono services are provided can be a difficult situation with regards to ethics and distribution of resources. PTs and/or PTAs should have delineated policies and procedures for establishing need and administering pro bono services.

DOCUMENTATION AND REIMBURSEMENT

In 1966, Medicare and Medicaid began requiring physicians and other health care providers to document medical procedures in order to be reimbursed.[27] In 1997, Baeten[28(p14)] indicated that documentation is the "key to securing reimbursement." Physical therapy documentation should include the physical therapist's initial examination, evaluation, and plan of care. Daily or treatment notes, progress notes, re-evaluations (as necessary), and a final discharge summary should follow the initial evaluation.

The primary documentation role of the PTA is writing daily notes. To maximize reimbursement, daily notes must do the following:

- Reflect a comparison between the patient's current functional status and his or her functional status at the initial evaluation.[29]
- Include impairments and functional deficits in clear, concise, objective, and measurable language.[29]
- Maximize the use of objective tests and measures and avoid terms such as *decreased strength*.[2,29]
- Describe the assistance provided and distinguish between verbal and physical assistance.[29]
- Include regular patient updates[29]; that is, tests and measurements (range of motion, strength) and functional status (gait, transfers, ADL, and IADL) should be provided throughout the record, not just on the evaluations and re-evaluations.
- Provide patient updates in a manner consistent with those on the initial evaluation[29]; that is, tests and measurements performed throughout the episode of care should be consistent with those performed during the initial examination.
- Indicate why progress might be slower than expected; for example, in the presence of comorbidities.[29]

- Provide adequate information to support medical necessity of each treatment/procedure on every date it was billed.[29]
- Provide evidence that unique services of a therapist (skilled services) are required. This includes recording patient's response to treatment and recommending a re-evaluation for changes to the treatment plan when necessary.[29]
- Include the time spent delivering each service.[29]
- Include a description of the service provided in language that is consistent with what is billed.[2,29]

When documenting, you should always keep in mind that payment could depend upon what you write in the progress notes. It is not enough to write "Pt. improving," "tolerated well," or "skilled services needed." Rather, describe changes in specific objective terms (ie, level of assist decreased from moderate assist to supervision; knee flexion increased 30°). Other key points you should always make include (1) the ongoing need for skilled interventions and (2) how those interventions bring about functional improvement.

REFERENCES

1. American Physical Therapy Association. Glossary of payment terms. Available at: http://www.apta.org/Payment/Glossary/. Accessed April 22, 2011.
2. American Physical Therapy Association. *The Reimbursement Resource Guide.* Alexandria, Va: American Physical Therapy Association; 2002.
3. Social Security Administration. History. Available at: http://www.ssa.gov/history/law.html. Accessed January 28, 2012.
4. Medicare. Medicare eligibility tool. Available at: http://www.medicare.gov/MedicareEligibility/Home.asp?dest=NAV|Home|GeneralEnrollment#TabTop. Accessed April 22, 2011.
5. U.S. Department of Health and Human Services. Remarks by HHS Secretary Tommy G. Thompson at Press Conference Announcing Reforming Medicare and Medicaid Agency [press release]. Available at: http://findarticles.com/p/articles/mi_m3257/is_8_55/ai_78363222/?tag=content;col1. Accessed January 28, 2012.
6. Centers for Medicare and Medicaid Services. What is CMS? Available at: http://questions.cms.hhs.gov/app/answers/detail/a_id/1. Accessed April 22, 2011.
7. Centers for Medicare and Medicaid Services. National CHIP policy: an overview. Available at: http://www.cms.gov/NationalCHIPPolicy/. Accessed April 22, 2011.
8. Centers for Medicare and Medicaid Services. Medicare and you 2011. Available at: http://www.medicare.gov/Publications/Pubs/pdf/10050.pdf. Accessed May 6, 2011.
9. Centers for Medicare and Medicaid Services. Medicare glossary. Available at: http://www.medicare.gov/Glossary/Search.asp. Accessed May 6, 2011.
10. Centers for Medicare and Medicaid Services. Prospective payment systems—general information. Available at: http://www.cms.gov/ProspMedicareFeeSvcPmtGen/. Accessed May 6, 2011.
11. Centers for Medicare and Medicaid Services. CMS glossary. Available at: http://www.cms.gov/apps/glossary/. Accessed May 6, 2011.
12. American Physical Therapy Association. Payment by treatment setting. Available at: http://www.apta.org/Payment/PrivateInsurance/PaymentbySetting/. Accessed May 17, 2011.
13. Centers for Medicare and Medicaid Services. Skilled nursing facility prospective payment system—an overview. Available at: http://www.cms.gov/SNFPPS/01_overview.asp. Accessed May 6, 2011.
14. Centers for Medicare and Medicaid Services. Inpatient rehab prospective payment system—an overview. Available at: http://www.cms.gov/InpatientRehabFacPPS/01_overview.asp. Accessed May 6, 2011.
15. Uniform Data System for Medical Rehabilitation. About the FIM system. Available at: http://www.udsmr.org/WebModules/FIM/FIM_About.aspx. Accessed January 28, 2012.
16. Centers for Medicare and Medicaid Services. Home health prospective payment system—an overview. Available at: http://www.cms.gov/HomeHealthPPS/01_overview.asp. Accessed May 6, 2011.
17. Centers for Medicare and Medicaid Services. Overview. Available at: http://www.cms.gov/apps/physician-fee-schedule/. Updated January 18, 2012. Accessed January 28, 2012.
18. American Medical Association. About CPT. Available at: http://www.ama-assn.org/ama/pub/physician-resources/solutions-managing-your-practice/coding-billing-insurance/cpt/about-cpt.page. Accessed January 28, 2012.
19. American Medical Association. RBRVS: Resource-Based Relative Value System. Available at: http://www.ama-assn.org/ama/pub/physician-resources/solutions-managing-your-practice/coding-billing-insurance/medicare/the-resource-based-relative-value-scale.page. Accessed January 28, 2012.
20. American Medical Association. The Medicare Physician Payment Schedule. Available at: http://www.ama-assn.org/ama/pub/physician-resources/solutions-managing-your-practice/coding-billing-insurance/medicare/the-medicare-physician-payment-schedule.page. Accessed January 28, 2012.
21. American Medical Association. CPT Code/Relative Value search. Available at: https://ocm.ama-assn.org/OCM/CPTRelativeValueSearch.do. Accessed January 28, 2012.
22. Centers for Medicare and Medicaid Services. *Medicaid-at-a-Glance.* Publication No. CMS-11024-05. Available at: http://www.cms.gov/MedicaidDataSourcesGenInfo/downloads/maag2005.pdf. Accessed May 17, 2011.
23. Centers for Medicare and Medicaid Services. Medicare claims processing manual. Available at: http://www.cms.gov/BNI/Downloads/RevABNManualInstructions.pdf. Accessed May 17, 2011.
24. Medline Plus. Managed care. Available at: http://www.nlm.nih.gov/medlineplus/managedcare.html. Accessed May 17, 2011.
25. Cohn R. Understanding insurance coverage. *PT Magazine.* 1999;7(10).
26. Elliott C. Responding to cost shifts. Available at: http://www.apta.org/PTinMotion/2009/5/GovernmentAffairs/. Accessed May 17, 2011.
27. Inaba M, Jones SL. Medical documentation for third-party payers. *Phys Ther.* 1977;57:791–794.
28. Baeten AM. Documentation: the reviewer perspective. *Top Geriatr Rehabil.* 1997;13(1):14–22.
29. United Government Services LLC. Best documentation: concise and complete. Presented at: Medicare Outpatient Therapy Services Educational Seminar; May 17, 2004.

Review Questions

1. In your own words, define reimbursement.

2. Who are the different parties responsible for the financial management of a patient's medical care? What is meant by third-party payment?

3. Describe the 4 types of insurance outlined here (social, managed care, casualty, and indemnity).

4. What are the major differences between Medicare Part A and Medicare Part B? What is Part C?

5. What is the difference between Medicare and Medicaid?

6. What strategies are used by managed care organizations to contain or lower costs? Give a brief description of each.

7. Define cash-based services. What are some advantages and disadvantages of cash-based services?

8. Talk with a local clinician about different types of insurance often accepted by their facility. What are their reimbursement guidelines? Try to get examples of managed care plans, Medicare, and Medicaid.

9. Describe pro bono. Describe a scenario where administering pro bono services can lead to ethical decision making.

10. Complete the following table.

Facility	Type of PPS	Patient Categorization	Assessment
A. Acute care hospital	_____	_____	_____
B. _____	_____	_____	OASIS
C. _____	_____	RUG	_____
D. Inpatient rehabilitation facility	_____	_____	_____

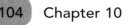

APPLICATION EXERCISE

I. Which of the following progress notes best meets the criteria for reimbursement? Why?

Note 1

S: Patient reporting improvement in her ability to wash her hair and dress with the left arm. Reports pain as 3/10 with excessive overhead activities and at night.

O: *AROM:* left shoulder flexion 130°, abduction 120°. Treatment consisted of 30 minutes of therapeutic exercises to increase shoulder range of motion, including 20 reps of wand exercises for flexion, external rotation, internal rotation, and abduction, manual stretching in the above directions, pulley for 5 minutes, and finger ladder for 5 minutes.

A: Exercises allowing improved ROM. AROM improved 45° since initial visit. Increased motion allowing improved self-care. Patient achieves greater manual stretch from therapist than through self-stretch.

P: Continue with above program with progression per plan of care as stated on initial eval.

Sally Smith, PTA

Note 2

S: Continues to report night pain and when reaching overhead.

O: Increased AROM; performed 30 minutes of active and passive exercises to improve joint range of motion.

A: Tolerated well.

P: Continue above 2x/week.

Sally Smith, PTA

Note 3

S: Patient complains of pain with excessive overhead activities and at night. Having trouble sleeping.

O: *AROM:* left shoulder flexion 130°, abduction 120°. Treatment consisted of 20 reps of wand exercises for flexion, external rotation, internal rotation, and abduction, manual stretching in the above directions, pulley for 5 minutes, and finger ladder for 5 minutes.

A: AROM improved since initial visit.

P: Continue with above program.

Sally Smith, PTA

Chapter 11

Legal and Ethical Considerations for Physical Therapy Documentation

Mia L. Erickson, PT, EdD, CHT, ATC

CHAPTER OBJECTIVES

After reading this chapter, the student will be able to do the following:

1. Describe federal legislation related to privacy and confidentiality.
2. Discuss clinic requirements under the Health Insurance Portability and Accountability Act (HIPAA) privacy rule.
3. Compare ethical and legal responsibilities for maintaining confidentiality.
4. Define *fraud* and *abuse*.
5. Explain the purpose of risk management.
6. Realize the importance of informed consent.
7. Give reasons for filing an incident report.
8. Outline different agencies' responsibilities in establishing rules for documentation.

INTRODUCTION

As previously indicated, documentation will be one of the most important aspects of your job. When individuals consider becoming a PT or PTA, they generally do not realize the documentation requirements or their importance. After being in practice for several years and treating a variety of patients, it will become impossible to recall details of each patient encounter. Therefore, the information you record while details are fresh in your head will be your reference material if ever necessary. You should document so that if you read the chart several years later you can recall the patient.

Though a full review of legal and ethical requirements and implications for medical record keeping is beyond the scope of this chapter, it should provide an overview of important legal and ethical matters relevant to physical therapy documentation that influence day-to-day PTA practice. These are patient privacy and confidentiality, fraud and abuse, and medical malpractice.

PATIENT PRIVACY AND CONFIDENTIALITY

The Privacy Act of 1974 (5USC §552a)

The Privacy Act of 1974[1] set forth federal guidelines precluding health care agencies or providers from releasing or disclosing medical records or medical information to any person without first obtaining written consent, or a written request, from the patient. The Privacy Act required providers and their employees to be trained on rules for handling an individual's records, and administrative efforts were aimed at minimizing threats to maintaining patient confidentiality. This legislation also allowed the patient the right to obtain a copy of his or her medical records (charges can be applied) and discuss the records with his or her provider in the presence of another individual of the patient's choosing. Failure to comply with this Privacy Act would result in civil action against the provider.

In a clinical environment, it is important to maintain and respect the privacy and confidentiality of all information related to patients and clients. When working, you should

Erickson M, McKnight R. *Documentation Basics:*
A Guide for the Physical Therapist Assistant, Second Edition (pp. 105-110)
© 2012 SLACK Incorporated

take care not to leave charts in open areas, accessible to people walking by, and you should be careful not to dictate in an open area where you can be heard by others. Charts should also be kept in a secure, locked location so they are not accessible to unauthorized individuals. Computer monitors should "time out" after a brief period of nonuse and should be accessible to employees only. Clinics and hospitals are also likely to have policies preventing you from taking medical records out of the building. Though the Privacy Act of 1974 still holds true today, additional legislation has been passed to further restrict release of an individual's health information and medical records, including those transmitted via electronic media.

Health Insurance Portability and Accountability Act

Though electronic transmission of information, including billing and claims filing, was meant to simplify some of these processes, it also increased the risks of violating patient privacy and breaching confidentiality. In response, congress mandated the Health Insurance Portability and Accountability Act (HIPAA) of 1996 (PL 104-191).[2] This legislation required the Department of Health and Human Services (DHHS) to implement standards for performing electronic health care transactions, ensuring patient privacy provisions, and protecting personally identifiable health information, or protected health information (PHI).[3] The DHHS provided regulations, known as the Privacy Rule and the Security Rule, in order to implement the HIPAA requirment.[4]

The Privacy Rule

The Privacy Rule standards addressed how covered entities use and disclose an individual's protected health information.[3] "A major goal of the Privacy Rule is to assure that individual's health information is properly protected while allowing the flow of health information needed to provide and promote high quality health care."[1(p1)]

Health care providers, health plans, and health care clearinghouses are considered "covered entities," subject to the rule if they transmit PHI through any type of media, including electronic, oral, written, or facsimile. Protected health information includes both personal health information and individually identifiable health information. Electronic media refers to the Internet, intranets and extranets, leased lines, dial-up lines, private networks, or transmissions occurring through magnetic tape, disk, or compact disk.[5] The standards apply to health care providers in both private and public sectors (ie, private and government-run hospitals); those who are and are not associated with an institution such as a hospital, including physical therapists; and those who transmit information directly or indirectly through a third party or billing source.[3]

In addition to protecting identifiable health information, the Privacy Rule requires providers to (1) make available to patients both written and posted explanations of privacy rights, (2) allow easier patient access to medical records (although charges may be applied), (3) provide employee privacy training, and (4) appoint a privacy officer. Under the Privacy Rule, however, providers are allowed to supply information to insurance companies and third-party payers when seeking reimbursement, and they are permitted to discuss information with other health care providers who are caring for the patient, without any additional written consent from the patient. Information provided to these entities should be on a minimum necessary basis, meaning that providers should only disclose the minimum necessary information relevant to accomplish the purpose.[5]

The Security Rule

The Security Rule was finalized after the Privacy Rule. It protects a subset of the protected health information listed in the Privacy Rule; that is, e-PHI or any protected health information held or transferred in an electronic format. In addition, it provides necessary physical and technical safeguards that must be put into place to protect e-PHI. These physical and technical safeguards include things like limiting access to facilities and workstations, altering and destroying e-PHI, and transmitting e-PHI.

HIPAA does not replace any state laws, nor does it preclude states from having more restrictive legislation for protecting patient privacy. HIPAA's Privacy Rule merely provides minimum acceptable standards for maintaining and protecting patient privacy.[5] You should investigate the privacy laws in your state as they may differ.

Privacy Recommendations and Computerized Documentation

Maintaining privacy and confidentiality of electronic medical records can be accomplished in several ways. For example, computer systems maintaining patient records must be password protected and secured to prevent unauthorized use and assure private transmittals. The American Medical Association recommends assigning different security levels to differing degrees of data sensitivity to limit who has access to the information.[6] Computer terminals should be in private areas. Laptops and tablets should be held or placed where they are not viewable by patients. Privacy screen filters can also be used. Computers should "time out" after a brief period of non-use. Finally, there must be a process for backing-up and storing records.[5,6]

Privacy and Ethics

It is important to understand the difference between ethical and legal responsibilities. Simply stated, ethical responsibility is generally determined by professional associations through development and implementation of a code of ethics. Legal responsibilities are determined by both state and federal laws, and failure to comply with the law can result in civil and/or criminal action. You should also realize that unethical behavior or conduct is not always illegal. On the other hand, illegal conduct is usually unethical. Your ethical responsibilities as a PTA have been identified in the *Standards of Ethical Conduct for the Physical Therapist Assistant*[7] and interpreted in the *Guide for Conduct for the Physical Therapist Assistant*.[8] Standard 2, Part D, indicates that PTAs shall protect confidential patient information and provide it only when appropriate and allowed by law (in collaboration with the PT).[7]

FRAUD AND ABUSE

Each year, Medicare and its beneficiaries pay millions of dollars toward fraudulent claims. Insurance fraud can be defined as intentionally billing an insurance company, Medicare, or other third-party payer for services that were never provided or billing for an item or service that has higher reimbursement than the service provided.[9] Insurance fraud is both illegal and unethical. It is a crime and is punishable by law. Medicare beneficiaries are encouraged to report suspected accounts of fraudulent activity to the Office of the Inspector General. The *Standards of Ethical Conduct for the Physical Therapist Assistant*[7] and the *Guide for Conduct for the Physical Therapist Assistant*[8] put forth that PTAs should demonstrate integrity, including providing truthful and accurate information and discouraging misconduct. Keeping with this responsibility, it is also the PTA's duty to report any unethical or illegal acts, including knowledge of fraudulent billing practices.[7,8]

Another improper billing procedure is abuse. Abuse is when a provider bills for items that are not covered or unknowingly misuses billing codes. Abuse occurs when doctors or suppliers do not follow good medical practices, which result in unnecessary costs, improper payment, or provision of services that are not medically necessary.[9] Abuse differs from fraud in that abuse is usually a result of an error or unawareness of the proper code(s) or coding procedure(s). The terms *fraud* and *abuse* are often used interchangeably; however, they are very different. You should stay informed of reimbursement guidelines for insurance companies or payers that you encounter frequently.

RISK MANAGEMENT

A growing concern in litigious times and societies is risk management. In this context, *risk* is defined as the possibility of becoming subject to a liability claim with resulting financial or professional loss(es).[10] Facilities are likely to have risk managers, or risk management departments or committees, whose responsibilities include minimizing potential risks for therapists (PTs and PTAs) who are involved with patient/client management. These individual(s) investigate complaints or concerns as they are brought forth, usually by patients. An important aspect of their investigation is examining the patient record and available documentation. The documentation allows the risk manager(s) to "determine if the care provided met the standard of care required of prudent health care providers."[10]

Two important risk management documents that PTAs should be aware of are informed consent documents and incident reports. *Informed consent* is when a patient agrees to or rejects a specified treatment after being provided with a clear, thorough explanation of its risks, benefits, and treatment alternatives, when available. Additionally, the patient must be provided with information on the probability of success of the treatment as well as the consequences of no treatment at all.[10,11] The PT is ethically responsible for obtaining informed consent prior to providing any intervention. However, the PTA might need to obtain informed consent if initiating a new modality or exercise, as instructed by the PT. Therefore, it is critical to be aware of the patient's previous medical history and current pathology. It is necessary to stay abreast of literature describing indications and contraindications of various interventions that you will be providing. You should be able to recognize and communicate contraindications to treatment to the supervising PT. In addition, you should be able to describe to patients the risks, benefits, and alternatives to interventions you perform.

An incident report is a document completed when there is an incident that could likely result in a lawsuit. The goal is to document incidents that occur that are unexpected and deviate from normal day-to-day operations.[12] A report prepared by the University of California at San Francisco outlined 3 categories of critical incidents needing to be recorded, should they occur. These categories include adverse outcomes to a treatment that has been provided, procedural breakdowns, and catastrophic events.[12] Examples in physical therapy include patients falling during gait training, accidental burns from hot packs or other modality, injuries sustained during therapeutic exercises, or any other event that has potential to harm a patient or visitor within or around the hospital or clinic. Incident reports are filed with the risk management department, not recorded in the patient's medical chart.

ESTABLISHING DOCUMENTATION REQUIREMENTS

Federal Agencies

The Centers for Medicare & Medicaid Services has set forth policies requiring health care facilities (inpatient, outpatient, and home health) seeking reimbursement from Medicare and Medicaid to maintain documentation to support services provided and billed. The most current documentation guidelines for Medicare can be found on the CMS Web site (www.cms.gov). They are available for inpatient rehabilitation facilities (Chapter 1), home health services (Chapters 8 and 9), skilled nursing facilities (Chapter 6), and outpatient facilities (Chapter 15).[13] However, these are CMS's requirements and can only be applied to Medicare and Medicaid. Nevertheless, private insurance companies or other reimbursing agencies can and have adopted similar requirements. In addition, the Joint Commission on Accreditation of Health Care Organizations (JCAHO) requires facilities that it accredits to maintain medical records for each patient.

State Practice Acts

Both PTs and PTAs are bound by practice acts in the state(s) where they provide care to patients. Each state has different provisions for PT and PTA practice, some more restrictive than others. The state practice acts may outline provisions for PTA documentation. The Federation of State Boards of Physical Therapy (FSBPT) has provided a Web site with links to state licensing agencies and state practice acts. This can be found at www.fsbpt.org/LicensingAuthorities/index.asp. You should become familiar with the practice act for any state where you provide elements of patient/client management.

American Physical Therapy Association

The APTA has published many recommendations for appropriate documentation. These include *Guidelines: Physical Therapy Documentation of Patient/Client Management*[14] and "Defensible Documentation,"[15] which have been referred to throughout this book.

Though the national association represents physical therapy practitioners across the country, it is important to point out that the documentation guidelines set forth by the APTA are only to serve as a guide. Physical therapy providers (PTs and PTAs) must be first and foremost in compliance with their state practice acts before implementing APTA recommendations. In addition, documentation requirements and guidelines are dynamic and tend to change as the scope of practice evolves. It is your professional responsibility to stay attuned to important changes in documentation requirements, and from a legal perspective, complying first to state laws where you practice is necessary to maintain licensure.

REFERENCES

1. The Privacy Act of 1974. 5USC §552a. Available at: http://www.justice.gov/oplc/privstat.htm. Updated September 26, 2003. Accessed January 29, 2012.
2. Health Insurance Portability and Accountability Act of 1996, PL 104-141. 104th Congress. Available at: http://hhs.gov/ocr/privacy/hipaa/administrative/statute/index.html. Published August 21, 1996. Accessed January 29, 2012.
3. US Department of Health and Human Services. OCR Privacy Rule summary. Available at: http://www.hhs.gov/ocr/privacy/hipaa/understanding/summary/privacysummary.pdf. Accessed May 18, 2011.
4. US Department of Health and Human Services. Summary of the HIPAA Security Rule. Available at: http://www.hhs.gov/ocr/privacy/hipaa/understanding/srsummary.html. Accessed May 18, 2011.
5. Ravitz KS. The HIPAA privacy final modified rule. *PT Magazine*. 2002;10(11):21-25
6. American Medical Association. AMA Opinions and Standards: 5.07 confidentiality: computers. Available at: http://www.netreach.net/~wmanning/ama507.htm. Accessed May 18, 2011.
7. American Physical Therapy Association House of Delegates. *Standards of Ethical Conduct for the Physical Therapist Assistant*. HOD 06-09-20-18. Available at: http://www.apta.org/uploadedFiles/APTAorg/About_Us/Policies/HOD/Ethics/Standards.pdf. Accessed May 18, 2011.
8. American Physical Therapy Association Ethics and Judicial Committee. *Guide for Conduct for the Physical Therapist Assistant*. Available at: http://www.apta.org/uploadedFiles/APTAorg/About_Us/Policies/Bylaws_and_Rules/GuidefortheConductofthePTA.pdf. Accessed May 18, 2011.
9. Centers for Medicare and Medicaid Services. Fraud and abuse. Available at: http://www.medicare.gov/navigation/help-and-support/fraud-and-abuse/fraud-and-abuse-overview.aspx. Accessed May 18, 2011.
10. Price SA. Risk management. Presented at: Annual Meeting of the West Virginia Physical Therapists' Association; August 9, 1997.
11. Smith LC. Risk management: the hot topics. *PT Magazine*. December 2000;8:26–33.
12. Agency for Healthcare Research and Quality. Making health care safer: a critical analysis of patient safety practices. Available at: http://www.ahrq.gov/clinic/ptsafety/. Accessed May 18, 2011.
13. Centers for Medicare and Medicaid Services. Internet-Only Manuals. Available at: http://www.cms.gov/Manuals/IOM/ItemDetail.asp?ItemID=CMS012673. Accessed January 29, 2012.
14. American Physical Therapy Association. *Guidelines: Physical Therapy Documentation of Patient/Client Management*. BOD: G03-05-16-41. Available at: http://www.apta.org/uploadedFiles/APTAorg/About_Us/Policies/BOD/Practice/DocumentationPatientClientMgmt.pdf. Accessed May 18, 2011.
15. American Physical Therapy Association. Defensible documentation. Available at: http://www.apta.org/Documentation/DefensibleDocumentation/. Accessed May 17, 2011.

REVIEW QUESTIONS

1. What guidelines did the Privacy Act of 1974 establish?

2. What was the rationale for developing the HIPAA Privacy and Security Rules?

3. What are the requirements for health care providers under the HIPAA Privacy and Security Rules?

4. How do HIPAA's Privacy and Security Rules affect state law?

5. What is your ethical responsibility regarding confidentiality and documentation? Is this different from your legal responsibility? Why or why not?

6. Differentiate between fraud and abuse. Give an example of each.

7. What are your ethical responsibilities related to fraud and abuse?

8. Define risk management.

9. What is the role of risk managers?

10. How is documentation important to risk managers?

11. When seeking informed consent from a patient, what are the key pieces of information that should be provided to the patient?

12. Give 3 examples (other than those listed in the text) of when a PTA would need to file an incident report.

13. What state and federal government agencies are responsible for setting guidelines for medical record documentation?

14. To what document(s) can you refer to find information regarding physical therapy documentation in your state?

15. Investigate the physical therapy practice act for documentation requirements in your state. How does it compare with the FSBPT's model practice act?

Chapter 12
SOAP Notes Across the Curriculum

Mia L. Erickson, PT, EdD, CHT, ATC

The goal of "SOAP Notes Across the Curriculum" (SNAC) is to provide you with more examples and practice. SNAC is organized by topics frequently covered in a PTA curriculum. This includes a variety of physical therapy content areas and settings. Each topic or section provides additional documentation examples for you to work through. There are examples that will only require you to rewrite a few pieces of information to make them suitable for entry into a medical record. There are examples where you will be given an entire treatment session and you will have to rewrite the information, creating an entire SOAP note. Finally, there are examples where you will have to come up with the A and/or P sections of the note based on the available information or after referring to the patient's initial note that has been provided. In all cases, you should write clearly and concisely, using appropriate abbreviations, symbols (Appendix A), and medical terminology. You can use this section all at once during the documentation unit or throughout your program as you cover the different content areas. Your instructor will guide you on how he or she wants you to complete this section.

The following physical therapy content areas are included in SNAC:
- Goniometry
- Strength assessment
- Therapeutic exercises
- Transfers
- Tilt table
- Wheelchair management
- Gait training
- Wound care
- Chronic obstructive pulmonary disease/vital signs
- Traumatic brain injury (TBI)
- Spinal cord injury (SCI)
- Cerebrovascular accident (CVA)
- Lower extremity amputation/prosthetic devices
- Musculoskeletal trauma
- Pediatrics/orthotic devices

GONIOMETRY

For each of the following, rewrite the information so that it would be appropriate for recording into a SOAP note. Include S, O, A, and P where appropriate.

1. You are working on increasing range of motion in a patient who had a right bimalleolar fracture. After taking the following measurements, you decide that her active range of motion goal has been met and she should be re-evaluated by the PT. Active range of motion on the right ankle was 10° dorsiflexion and 50° plantarflexion. The left has 15° dorsiflexion and 55° plantarflexion.

2. You take the following measurements from a patient who is 3 weeks' status post-right cerebrovascular accident with left hemiplegia. Active range of motion on the right upper and lower extremities is within normal limits. However, on the left, active range of motion is decreased, including shoulder: 45° flexion and abduction, 40° internal rotation, 60° external rotation; elbow: flexion 100° and extension 0°; wrist extension 0° and flexion 50°. For the left

Erickson M, McKnight R. *Documentation Basics: A Guide for the Physical Therapist Assistant, Second Edition* (pp. 111-126)
© 2012 SLACK Incorporated

lower extremity, hip: flexion 120°, abduction 20°; knee flexion 130° and extension 0°; ankle dorsiflexion 0° and plantarflexion 50°.

3. The following measurements were taken from a patient on 6/21/11. Active range of motion: right wrist flexion 50°, extension 60°, supination 45°, pronation 45°, ulnar deviation 10°, and radial deviation 5°. On 6/24, you record the following measurements for the same patient. Active range of motion: right wrist flexion 62°, extension 65°, supination 55°, pronation 60°, ulnar deviation 15°, and radial deviation 10°. Organize the measurements for the note on 6/24. Also, what would your assessment be for that day?

4. You are working with a patient who has multiple sclerosis. You record the following measurements. Active range of motion measurements taken at the ankles: 0° dorsiflexion and 50° plantarflexion, at the knees: extension −20° and flexion 135°, at the hips: flexion 100°, and abduction 20°. Passive range of motion measurements: ankles: 20° dorsiflexion, knees: 0° extension, and hips: 120° flexion.

STRENGTH ASSESSMENT

Rewrite the following information so that it would be appropriate for recording into a SOAP note. You will need to assign the appropriate muscle grade(s) based on the description provided.

Your supervising PT has asked you to perform manual muscle testing on a patient. Your findings are below.

1. When assessing the patient's right upper extremity, he is able to take moderate to strong resistance in all muscle groups except abduction and lateral rotation where he is only able to take moderate resistance. Also, he is able to take strong resistance with elbow extension. All muscle tests were performed in the antigravity position.

2. When assessing the patient's right lower extremity, he is able to take slight resistance with hip abduction; slight to moderate resistance with hip flexion, hip extension, and hip lateral rotation; moderate resistance with knee flexion; moderate to strong resistance with hip adduction, knee extension, and ankle dorsiflexion; and strong resistance with ankle plantarflexion. All muscle tests were performed in the antigravity position.

3. When assessing the patient's left upper extremity, you must use the gravity-eliminated position for all testing. The patient is able to complete full range in this position (he is only able to complete 25% of the range in the gravity-resisted position) and takes some resistance for shoulder adduction and medial rotation. The patient is only able to move through approximately 50% of the available range

of motion in the gravity-eliminated position when testing shoulder flexion, shoulder extension, shoulder abduction, and elbow extension. The patient is able to complete full available range of motion in the gravity-eliminated position for elbow flexion. You are only able to palpate contractions for the shoulder lateral rotators and the wrist flexors and extensors in the gravity eliminated positions.

4. When assessing the patient's left lower extremity, he was able to take slight resistance in the antigravity position when testing hip extensors, hip adductors, and hip internal rotators. He was able to complete full active range of motion and maintain the test position against gravity for hip flexors and ankle plantarflexors. He was unable to complete full range of motion against gravity with hip lateral rotators and knee extensors. He was able to complete only 50% of available range of motion in the gravity-eliminated position for the hip abductors. Only a palpable contraction could be noted with knee flexors and ankle dorsiflexors.

THERAPEUTIC EXERCISES

1. Organize the following 3 cases into SOAP format.

Case 1. You are working in the acute hospital setting with an elderly female who has suffered a right CVA. The supervising therapist has asked you to assist with part of this patient's therapy today. The patient is cooperative and has no complaints. You performed passive and active assisted range of motion to the patient's left extremities. The patient was not showing any signs of abnormal tone or signs of developing contractures. You performed 3 sets of 10 repetitions. You also provided manual resistance to the patient's right lower extremity in proprioceptive neuromuscular facilitation (PNF) D1 and D2 patterns. The patient tolerated 2 sets of 10 repetitions for the resisted range of motion. Finally, you provided stretching to the patient's tight ankle plantarflexors bilaterally. You provided the stretch 5 times for each side holding each stretch for 30 seconds. You will continue the same treatment the following day and progress as instructed by the PT. The treatment session lasted 12'.

Case 2. You just finished working with a patient receiving home health care who had a total knee arthroplasty 10 days ago. She was in her bed and performed exercises to work on range of motion. She said she had some pain during the previous night, and she continues to have swelling that she feels is preventing her from bending her knee more. Her biggest complaints right now are not being able to sit normally, go up and down stairs, or drive due to the range of motion limitations in the knee. Her active motion at the knee was 10° extension and 95° flexion. You had the patient perform 20 repetitions of heel slides, ankle dorsiflexion and plantar flexion, short arc *knee extension exercises, and active hip abduction and adduction. You also worked on active-assistive range of motion to improve knee flexion while the patient was seated at the edge of the bed. She ambulated 50' times 2 with close supervision for balance and verbal cues for walker placement and sequencing, weight bearing as tolerated on the right with a standard walker. She stated that she felt good after the exercises. You tell her that you will see her in 2 days to continue the exercises and progress them as she can tolerate. Active knee motion increased to 110° following the treatment and he could sit more comfortably. Total treatment time was 45'.*

Case 3. You are working with a patient who had a rotator cuff repair 8 weeks ago. During the last session, you initiated resistive range of motion exercises (isometric setting) to begin strengthening the deltoid. He returns to the clinic today and tells you that he has felt good since his last treatment and thinks that the isometric exercises are getting too easy. He thinks that he is able to dress and perform self-care with greater ease. He also notes improved ability to reach into overhead cabinets. After consulting the plan of care, you decide to progress the patient to using an exercise band (2 sets of 10 repetitions). While in the clinic that day, he begins shoulder flexion and internal and external rotation using the yellow exercise band. He also performs his usual routine including 20 repetitions of flexion and external rotation with a wand, scapular retraction and protraction, and active external and internal rotation in the side lying position. You also perform 20 repetitions of passive range of motion for flexion, internal and external rotation, and abduction. After the treatment, he said he felt good and thought the new exercises were not that hard. He will return next week, and his exercises will be progressed per the rotator cuff protocol and as he is able to tolerate. Total treatment time was 45'.

2. From the 3 cases above, what pieces of information help you in determining the patient's response to the intervention?

3. Where would this response be documented in the note?

4. In your notes, did you describe the need for skilled services? How?

5. In your notes, did you link impairment to function (ie, activity limitations and participation restrictions)? How?

TRANSFERS

For each of the following, rewrite the information so that it would be appropriate for recording into a SOAP note.

1. The patient moved from the bed to the chair with 25% assistance provided by 1 therapist. The stand pivot transfer was used.

2. The patient moved from the wheelchair to the floor using both of his upper extremities with verbal cuing from the therapist.

3. The therapist transferred the patient in the Hoyer lift from the bed to the wheelchair.

4. The patient moved supine to sit and sit to supine with 50% of the assistance provided by the therapist.

5. The patient required 50% of the therapist's assistance when moving from the wheelchair to the mat table when transferring to the left (squat pivot transfer); however, she could transfer to the right with only 25% of assistance provided by the therapist.

6. Your client is a 58-year-old female who has suffered a compound fracture of the (R) ankle 2 days ago. You are to teach her how to transfer effectively from the wheelchair to the bedside commode. She is non-weight-bearing (NWB) on the affected side and is wearing a plaster cast, immobilizing the foot and ankle. The patient is obese and requires moderate assist of 2 people for transferring in and out of bed to a wheelchair. She says that she is in severe pain and is hesitant to participate. While using a walker, she was able to stand and doff her pants with minimal assistance but still required moderate assistance of 2 people to complete the transfer from the bed to the bedside commode due to fear of falling and difficulty maintaining NWB status.

7. You are working with a 68-year-old female who is recovering from a brainstem CVA. Slideboard transfer training with this patient has not gone well. The patient has made poor progress over the last 2 weeks, and the focus of treatment has changed to educating the husband on how to care for his wife. The supervising therapist has asked you to begin Hoyer transfer training with the patient and her husband. The patient is disappointed that she has not made any significant improvements, but she continues to be motivated and upbeat with therapy. She has stated that she is "not going to give up." The husband required moderate assistance placing the Hoyer sling and setting up for the transfer and needed minimal assistance during the transfer. The patient will be discharged to home with her husband as soon as he is able to care for her independently.

8. You are working with a 28-year-old patient who is in rehab due to a T4 SCI with paraplegia. During this therapy session, you concentrated on working with the patient on his slideboard transfers for 30'. The patient was able to perform wheelchair setup with minimal assistance of one to assist with weight shift and occasional verbal cues, but he required moderate assistance with slideboard placement. The

patient required maximal assistance with the transfer. The patient shared with you during therapy today that he is concerned about his family and how he was going to manage caring for the farm. The patient appeared depressed and anxious during this session. While looking at the initial evaluative note, you notice there is a goal for the patient to be independent in slideboard transfers.

9. You are working with an inpatient with Guillain Barré syndrome. He reports that he is doing better today. Exercises (3 sets of 10 reps) consisted of ankle pumps, active hip abduction, heel slides, bridging, and knee extension at the edge of the bed. After exercises, you worked on transfers to the wheelchair, which was positioned next to the bed using a stand pivot transfer. The patient required about 25%–30% assistance from you, but you were able to provide this yourself without difficulty, although you did have to block his knees so they did not buckle due to weakness. After this, the patient transferred back to bed, but because of fatigue and bed height, he requires 50%–60% assistance. He performed sit to and from supine with 50% assistance because of weakness. He was unable to lift his legs onto the bed from the floor. He was able to position himself in bed without the use of side rails while scooting and bridging with verbal cues. There was no improvement in the patient's ability to transfer from the previous day's note. You tell him you will see him in the afternoon for gait in the therapy department.

Tilt Table

For each of the following, rewrite the information so that it would be appropriate for recording into a SOAP note.

1. You are helping a 78-year-old patient who requires maximum assist from 3 to 4 people to stand. The therapist decides to begin standing activities on the tilt table. The patient has been sitting up in a wheelchair without any complaints or problems. The patient is able to tolerate getting to a full upright position and stay for 10 minutes before complaining of fatigue. The patient's blood pressure (BP) readings remained 120/74 for the full 10 minutes.

2. You are working with a 28-year-old patient who has a closed head injury and exhibits severe hypertonia. The therapist tells you to use the tilt table to help manage lower extremity spasticity. The patient tolerates the procedure without a change in BP (110/76). The patient remains in the upright position for 20 minutes.

3. A 67 year old who is recovering from a lengthy illness associated with acute respiratory failure is having consistent problems with orthostatic hypo-

tension. The patient has had 2 previous tilt table treatments and was able to get up to approximately 45° before her BP dropped significantly. At 0° it was 108/68. At 45° it was 92/58 after 1 minute.

Wheelchair Management

For each of the following, rewrite the information so that it would be appropriate for recording into a SOAP note.

1. The patient worked on wheelchair propulsion on ramps and level surfaces for 30 minutes, including tile and carpet, and he is now able to propel independently on all surfaces and manage leg rests and brakes without cuing.

2. You are working with a 16-year-old patient with a T1 spinal cord lesion. The patient currently needs moderate assistance to perform transfers to and from the wheelchair with a slideboard. The patient currently requires occasional verbal cues (v/c) and minimal assistance to set up the slideboard and prepare the wheelchair's arm and leg rests for safe mobility in and out.

3. The patient is 24 year old and was involved in a motor vehicle accident (MVA) and sustained bilateral femur fractures. The patient has undergone bilateral ORIFs and is now being taught slideboard transfers from the wheelchair to and from the bed. The patient requires moderate assistance for board setup and minimal assistance for managing the wheelchair parts. She needs moderate assistance from 2 people to transfer in and out of the wheelchair.

4. You are working with a 58-year-old patient with diabetes, a right above-knee amputation (AKA), and a left below-knee amputation (BKA). The patient has been assigned the following FIM[1] scores. Write the objective portion of your note so that levels of assistance correspond with the FIM scores. Bed, chair, and wheelchair transfers = 3; toilet, tub, and shower transfers = 2; wheelchair mobility = 4.

5. You are working with a patient who has a T3 complete spinal cord lesion with resultant paraplegia. He has been working on the slideboard to transfer in and out of his wheelchair. Currently he is requiring minimal assistant from the therapist (you) to set up and prepare the chair. He requires moderate assistance for the transfer. The ultimate goal is that he will be independent. You spend about 20 minutes on transfer training. He has also been working on wheelchair mobility, including ramps, gravel, sidewalks, and carpet. He can perform all of these mobility skills with verbal cuing for weight shifting and occasional minimal assist for trunk control. The goal for wheelchair mobility is also for independence (an additional 10 minutes is spent on

wheelchair mobility). For the last part of the treatment session (20 minutes) you work on transferring from the wheelchair to the floor. He requires minimal assist to go to the floor but requires maximal assist to get back into the chair. This goal is also for him to be independent. You notice on the initial evaluative note that the patient required maximal assist of 2 people for all transfers and moderate assist of 1 person for wheelchair mobility skills when he was admitted to the facility. The plan is to see him twice a day—in the morning for the above and in the afternoon for strengthening, stretching, and continued functional mobility.

GAIT TRAINING

For each of the following, rewrite the information so that it would be appropriate for recording into a SOAP note.

Parallel Bars

1. You are to help a 76-year-old obese patient who underwent bilateral total knee arthroplasties to ambulate in the parallel bars. She is able to ambulate 10' with moderate assistance of 1 person.
2. An 82-year-old patient with a right BKA is beginning gait training with his new prosthesis in the parallel bars. He is able to ambulate 20' with minimal assistance of 1 person. He required verbal cues to weight shift to the right.
3. A 45-year-old patient with multiple sclerosis has bilateral lower extremity weakness, coordination problems, and balance deficits ambulates 20' in the parallel bars with moderate assistance from 1 person and verbal cuing for upright posture.

Crutches

1. You are to assist a 46-year-old patient who underwent an arthroscopic surgery on his left lower extremity to ambulate with crutches. He is allowed to weight bear as tolerated and needs minimal assistance from 1 person for ambulation on level surfaces (for 30 feet) and up and down 2 steps.
2. You are assisting a 26-year-old patient who suffered a right femur fracture to ambulate with crutches. The patient is non-weight-bearing on the right lower extremity. The patient has poor balance but only requires minimal assistance from 1 person on level surfaces and up and down steps. The patient can ambulate for 50 feet before requiring a rest break.
3. You are working with a 38-year-old patient with multiple sclerosis who recently underwent a right total knee arthroplasty (TKA). The patient has

used Loftstrand crutches for years. You are assisting the patient in ambulating with the Loftstrand crutches. The patient requires moderate assistance and is allowed to weight bear as tolerated. She can ambulate 25 feet before requiring a break due to fatigue. She has considerably decreased endurance and becomes short of breath easily. Respiratory rate increased from 15 to 25 resp/min after gait.

Cane

1. You are assisting a 64-year-old patient with right CVA to ambulate with a hemi-cane. The patient requires moderate assistance from 1 person to ambulate 50'. She requires this assistance to advance her left leg.
2. You are assisting a 78-year-old patient who suffered a left humerus fracture and is having some mild balance deficits in learning to ambulate with a straight cane. The patient requires minimal assist of 1 person due to balance deficits to ambulate 150'.
3. A 64-year-old patient who underwent a right total hip arthroplasty 6 weeks ago is ready to advance from using a walker to using a cane. After instructing the patient to use a cane, you decided that he required contact guard assistance of 1 person and verbal cuing for proper sequencing to ambulate 75'.

Walker

1. You are assisting a 74-year-old patient who recently underwent a right total hip arthroplasty in learning how to ambulate with a walker. The patient requires moderate assistance of 1 person and is allowed to weight bear as tolerated to walk 75 feet.
2. You are assisting an 84-year-old patient who fell and suffered a right wrist and right femur fracture. The patient underwent an ORIF surgery and is partial weight-bearing on the right. You are to assist her in ambulating with a right platform walker. She requires moderate assistance for 25 feet and reminders that she can only place 50% of her weight on the involved lower extremity.
3. You are assisting an 88-year-old patient who is recovering from pneumonia. She is deconditioned and has mild balance problems. Her endurance is poor, so she is only able to ambulate 25' before tiring and requiring a rest break. The patient only requires minimal assistance and uses a wheeled walker. Her rate of perceived exertion was 17.

Organize the following 3 cases into SOAP format and then answer the questions that follow.

Case 1. You are assisting a 28-year-old male who underwent an open reduction internal fixation surgery for a fractured femur now weight bearing as tolerated on the right. You are assisting this patient with crutch gait on level surfaces and steps for 30'. The patient ambulates 300' on level surfaces and up and down 2 flights of steps independently and safely. The patient is ready for discharge. He voices that he wants to go home and is confident he will be able to handle himself. You reference the initial evaluation and note the patient has met all the goals established by the PT. He will be discharged to home in the next 1 to 2 days, and you think that home health would be a good idea for this patient.

Case 2. You are working with a 67 year old who underwent a left total hip replacement. You see the patient 2 days after the initial evaluation in the skilled nursing facility. Today the patient walked with the walker 100 feet on a level surface and only required contact guard assist from 1 person. At the time of the initial evaluation, the patient needed minimal assistance. You also began stair training. The patient walked up and down 5 steps with the rail and the walker and required constant verbal cues for sequencing and minimal assistance. The patient voices that he feels he is ready to go home. The goals are for the patient to be independent with gait 200 feet and on stairs since he will be home alone. You will continue to work on advancing him in gait and stairs so that he can return home.

Case 3. You have been working with a 72-year-old male who is recovering from a left CVA. The patient has improved his balance to the point that you are now working on gait in the parallel bars. The patient gets easily fatigued and is only able to take 5 to 6 steps at a time. The patient requires maximal assistance to ambulate and needs assistance advancing and placing his right leg. The patient voices that he is sure he will never be able to walk again and says, "We are wasting our time."

1. From the 3 cases above, what pieces of information help you in determining the patient's response to the intervention?
2. Where would this response be documented in the note?
3. In your notes, did you describe the need for skilled services? How?
4. In your notes, is your clinical problem solving apparent? Why or why not?
5. In your notes, did you link impairment to function (ie, activity limitations and participation restrictions)? How?

WOUND CARE

For each of the following, rewrite the information so that it would be appropriate for recording into a SOAP note.

1. Upon removing the dressing, you notice minimal drainage on the dressing. The drainage there is yellow exudate.
2. The wound bed is necrotic and is entirely filled with black eschar.
3. The area around the wound is red. It also feels warm. It is shiny, and there is also no hair around the wound.
4. After removing the previous day's dressing you notice a "sweet" odor and a moderate amount of greenish drainage on the dressing.
5. Wound is 4 cm in length and 2 cm in width. The depth is 3 mm. There is tunneling 2 inches at 12:00, toward the head.
6. The wound is located at the distal aspect of the right lateral leg, just below the lateral malleolus. It has a moderate amount of reddish brown drainage. It is 2 cm by 2 cm with no significant depth.
7. The wound is located on the top of the right foot. Edema is present in the foot and ankle. Figure 8 girth at the ankle is 20 cm on the right and 16 cm on the left. The periwound area is painful, red, and warm to the touch. The dorsal pedal pulse is present and is 1+ on the right and 2+ on the left.
8. The wound is on the anterior aspect of the left tibia. It is 3 cm in length and 4 cm in width. The depth is 5 mm. The wound is full thickness and irregularly shaped. It has 50% granulation and ~25% yellow slough. Part of the tibia and anterior tibialis are exposed. There is no odor present. Sensation is decreased to light touch on the left from the knee down. The treatment consisted of a warm water soak for 10' and dressing change using a hydrocolloid dressing to cover the wound.

Organize the following information into SOAP format.

You have been assigned a patient with a diagnosis of Stage 3 open wound at the head of the right first metatarsal, atherosclerosis, and diabetes mellitus. The patient complains of severe pain and has difficulty walking. There is a minimal amount of nonmalodorous reddish brown drainage from the wound bed. The wound bed is moist and has ~50% granulation tissue and 50% yellow adhered slough. The skin around the wound is red, warm to the touch, shiny, and swollen. The wound is a 4 cm × 2.4 cm oval-shaped wound. It is 1.5 cm deep. She has diminished sensation to light touch when compared bilateral. She is unable to feel the 10g monofilament on the right. Girth at the right metatarsophalangeal (MTP) joints is 22 cm and 18 cm on the left. The right dorsal pedis pulse is present but diminished compared to the left, which is 2+. Treatment consisted of whirlpool (WP) at 98°F × 15" to right lower extremity (LE) followed by debridement of a minimal amount of yellow slough from wound bed. After the treatment, the wound was covered with saline-soaked gauze and wrapped with Kling. It appears to you that the amount of yellow slough in the wound bed is decreasing. The initial evaluative note states that there was ~75% yellow adhered slough when the patient began the episode of care, although there is not much change in wound size. The plan is to continue with the above treatment and try to have the patient begin ambulating as she is able to tolerate.

CHRONIC OBSTRUCTIVE PULMONARY DISEASE/VITAL SIGNS

Organize the following information into SOAP format. Determine what to include in the A and P portions of the note. Try to incorporate evidence of the need for skilled care and link impairment to function, response to interventions, and clinical problem solving. After writing the note, consider what additional information you could include that would improve your note.

You have been assigned a 74-year-old female who is deconditioned with a diagnosis of chronic obstructive pulmonary disease. The treatment plan from the evaluative note (performed yesterday) states that the patient will be seen twice daily for endurance exercises and gait training. Upon entering the room, the patient is holding an oxygen mask to her face and taking deep inspirations and short expirations. She complains of difficulty breathing and moving around because she "can't get her breath." She is on 8 L of oxygen (O_2) at rest. Vital signs check before activity reveals the following: pulse 98 beats per minute (bpm), BP 120/84, respirations 20 per minute, O_2 saturation (SaO_2) 92%. She agrees to participate in bedside exercise, and you spend 15 minutes working on her upper and lower extremity AROM, assuring that her SaO_2 levels stay above 90%. After a rest break, she ambulates 30 feet from her bed to and from the bathroom with contact guard assist for safety. She requires the O_2 mask with oxygen levels set at 8 L during gait. She requires supervision during toileting secondary to complaints of dizziness. She returns to her bed and transfers sit to supine with moderate assist. After exercises and gait, her vitals are as follows: pulse 108 bpm, BP 124/84, respirations 24 per minute, SaO_2 90%. During the initial examination/evaluation, the patient was unable to ambulate because of her shortness of breath, and her resting vitals were as follows: pulse 104 bpm, BP 120/88, respirations 24 per minute, SaO_2 90% at rest.

TRAUMATIC BRAIN INJURY

Provided by Tracy Rice, PT, MPH, NCS

Organize the following information into SOAP format. Determine what to include in the A and P portions of the note. Try to incorporate evidence of the need for skilled care and link impairment to function, response to interventions, and clinical problem solving. After writing the note, consider what additional information could you include that would improve your note.

Your patient is a 17-year-old male in an inpatient rehabilitation facility. His diagnosis is diffuse axonal injury secondary to being ejected in a MVA. He presents with left-side weakness, increased tone, and spasticity. The patient presents with extensor tone/pattern on the left lower extremity and flexor tone/synergy on the left upper extremity. He is alert, awake, and inconsistently cooperative. He is oriented to person only. He is unaware of his situation, time, or place. He inconsistently follows simple commands, is sometimes combative, and demonstrates a short attention span. He responds well to an established routine and automatic tasks. His treatment session consisted of the following activities. You worked on bed mobility in the patient's room. He performed rolling to the right with moderate assistance x 1 and rolling to the left with minimal assistance x 1 and the use of the bed rail. The patient performed supine to sit at the edge of the bed (EOB) with moderate assistance x 1 and minimal assistance x 1 to maintain static sitting balance on the compliant bed surface. All bed mobility activities required verbal cues for sequencing. The patient performed a stand pivot transfer to the right from the bed to the wheelchair with moderate assistance x 1 and blocking of the left knee to prevent buckling. The patient propelled himself utilizing the right hemi-body to the therapy gym with verbal cues for sequencing the use of the wheelchair with the right upper extremity (UE) and LE and for attention to task. In the gym, you worked on additional functional activities. The patient performed wheelchair-to-mat transfer to the left with maximal assistance via stand pivot with blocking of the left knee to promote extension and prevent buckling. The patient performed repetitive sit to stand from the mat table with moderate assistance x 1 with manual assistance at the left LE for extension during the sit-to-stand transition. The patient ambulated 50' with rollator platform front-wheeled walker with minimal assistance of 1 to support the left UE and to guide the rollator and maximal assistance of another for manual assistance for step initiation on the left, blocking of left knee during stance phase of gait and for postural control as well. The patient required verbal cues throughout the gait process for upright posture, both head and trunk control, attention to task, and to increase step on the right LE to encourage stance on the left LE. The patient required his left ankle to be ace wrapped into dorsiflexion secondary to extensor tone and foot drop. He tolerated the standing frame for 45 minutes where you performed passive range of motion (PROM) to the left UE. You performed PROM to the shoulder in all planes of movement, the elbow, wrist, and hand, where you emphasized long finger extensors and increasing the web space and thumb abduction. Overall you feel that the patient is progressing and meeting his goals but continue to feel that he would benefit from inpatient acute rehabilitation.

SPINAL CORD INJURY

Provided by Tracy Rice, PT, MPH, NCS

Organize the following information into SOAP format. Determine what to include in the A and P portions of the note. Try to incorporate evidence of the need for skilled care and link impairment to function, response to interventions, and clinical problem solving. After writing the note, consider what additional information could you include that would improve your note.

Your patient is a 21-year-old with a T6 complete SCI as a result of an MVA. The patient is alert and oriented to person, place, time, and situation. He has been in acute rehabilitation for the last 2 weeks. He is making good progress and today his treatment consists of transfer training and functional activities in preparation for discharge to home. The patient performs repetitive wheelchair-to-mat and mat-to-wheelchair transfers. The patient performs them via multiple techniques to determine the most efficient and safest transfer technique as well as for functional endurance and strength training. The patient performs the transfer via lateral scoot with very close supervision to contact guard assist for wheel clearance. He performs that transfer repetitively x 5. Throughout the transfer sequence, the patient required verbal cues for technique. Verbal cues for scooting further forward in the chair, emphasizing the head–hip relationship, greater push through the UEs for better clearance, leaning forward and foot placement. He also performed wheelchair-to-mat and mat-to-wheelchair utilizing the transfer board with supervision and verbal cues for technique for board placement, head–hip relationship, and scooting with clearance rather than sliding on the board to protect his skin integrity. This technique was repeated 5 times. The patient performed short sitting on the edge of mat with supervision. The patient worked on dynamic sitting balance activities to encourage moving center of gravity over base of support: ball tossing, batting a balloon, reaching to the floor to don and doff shoes. All balance activities performed for 15 minutes as an endurance activity with close supervision to occasional contact guard assist for loss of balance. The patient performed sit to supine with supervision with for sequencing technique for efficiency. Once the patient was in supine, he worked on rolling left and right with supervision and verbal cues for technique with UE momentum and LE positioning. Worked on supine to long sitting with contact guard assist x 1 and verbal cues to maintain body weight anteriorly during the transition and then to prop self up on extended arms. Performed dynamic balance activities in long sitting to promote unsupported sitting without the use of bilateral UEs to allow for independent dressing. The patient performed ball tossing, batting a balloon, and lower body

(LB) dressing to promote moving center of gravity over base of support in long sitting. The patient transitioned to ring sitting and performed the same balance activities to promote independent sitting and independent self-care. The patient transitioned from ring sitting into prone lying with minimal assistance for LE management. From prone lying, the patient transitioned into side lying and then into sitting on the edge of the mat with minimal assistance and verbal cues for sequencing through the transitions. The therapy session ended by transferring from edge of mat to wheelchair via lateral scoot with contact guard assist x 1. The patient demonstrated good motivation and cooperation throughout the session despite having expressed some feelings of depression and longing to go home. His affect throughout is slightly flat, but he continues to be motivated and perform all activities asked of him despite the difficulty. Based on the treatment session you feel that the patient needs to continue to work on his transfer technique secondary to some technique flaws resulting in inefficiencies and not always clearing the surface in which he is transferring to, which places him at risk for skin breakdown.

CEREBROVASCULAR ACCIDENT

The following is an initial examination/evaluation for a patient recently admitted to an inpatient rehabilitation hospital. Use it to help you complete the following 2 SOAP notes. Include the following in your notes:

- Write the A and P portions of the notes based on available information here and in the evaluative notes.
- Write your notes to maximize reimbursement.
- Be specific when documenting your interventions (patient education, coordination or communication with other disciplines, and procedural intervention).
- What would be appropriate based on the plan of care provided and the patient's status?
- What would be corresponding FIM scores for this patient at the 2 points described above?

Pr: (L) CVA with (R) hemiparesis 1 week ago

Hx: 42 y.o. female admitted with sudden onset slurred speech, right facial droop, and right UE and LE weakness. The patient's PMH includes the long-term use of birth control and HTN, which is uncontrolled. She has had a mild CVA in the past affecting the left side of the body, but there are no residual impairments.

S: The patient states that she is having difficulty moving the right side of her body, the right UE more so than the right LE. She reports weakness in the right UE and LE. *PLOF*: Independent with all functional mobility and ADL without an assistive device. She worked full-time as a home health aide, drives, and takes care of her 7-year-old son. She is active in her child's activities and is also a volunteer in her community fire department. She is right-hand dominant. *Home Situation*: She lives alone with her 7-year-old son in a split-entry home with 4–5 steps with a unilateral handrail to both the first and second levels of the home. Her parents do live close by and are supportive. They are in good health and are able to assist as needed.

O: *Observation:* 3+ Pitting edema in right hand, decreased awareness of the right UE in general, and right facial droop with mild difficulty managing secretions.

Sensation: Impaired light touch, deep pressure, proprioception and kinesthesia to the right UE and LE but more so in the right UE.

Tone: The patient presents with decreased tone (hypotonia) with diminished reflexes 1+ throughout the right UE. Presents with increased extensor tone in the right LE, especially quadriceps, adductors, and plantarflexors. Modified Ashworth Scale (MAS)[2] score for the right quads, adductors, and plantarflexors is 2.

MMT: Left UE and LE 5/5 throughout.

Right UE grossly 1/5 throughout all shoulder musculature, 0/5 elbow, forearm, hand, and wrist.

Right LE: hip flexors = 2/5, quads = 2+/5, abductors 1+/5, adductors 2+/5, hamstrings 2–/5, PF = 2/5, DF = 0/5.

Functional Mobility:

Bed Mobility: The patient requires moderate assistance of 1 for rolling left, minimal assistance of 1 and the use of the bed rail for rolling to the right. Scooting in bed with moderate to maximal assistance of 1. The patient requires maximal assistance of 1 for supine to sit coming up on the right and moderate assistance for coming up on the left.

Transfers: Sit to stand from edge of bed with moderate assistance x 1 with blocking of right knee to prevent buckling and for stabilization and for postural control and balance. Sit to stand out of w/c with maximal assistance and the same stabilization required, greater assist required secondary to surface height difference. Bed to w/c transfers via stand pivot with moderate to maximal assistance of 1 depending on the surface height in which transferring and direction in which transferring. Requires right knee to be blocked for stabilization and to prevent buckling.

Gait: The patient ambulated 20' along left handrail in hallway with maximal assistance x 1 and a close follow with the w/c. The patient required the right ankle to be ace wrapped into DF and slight eversion secondary to foot drop and the inability to clear the foot during swing. The patient required manual assistance to complete swing, initiate the next step, and stabilize at the knee during stance to prevent buckling, shift weight, and assist at the pelvis to prevent pelvic retraction on the right.

Balance: Static sitting with minimal to moderate assistance depending on the compliance of the surface, static standing with maximal assistance, dynamic sitting with maximal assistance for moving center of gravity over base of support to the right more so than the left, dynamic standing with maximal assistance to dependent assistance.

Endurance: Fair, able to tolerate and complete the 1-hour evaluation session with 1 rest break every 10–15 minutes.

A: This is a 42 y.o. female with the diagnosis of a left CVA with right hemiparesis. The patient is currently unable to perform basic functional mobility or ADLs without at least moderate assistance. She is currently unable to care for herself or her 7-year-old son. Her prognosis is good for goals as stated and she would greatly benefit from inpatient acute rehabilitation for aggressive multidisciplinary services to meet her goals of returning home and therapy services to improve strength, balance, and functional mobility.

Problem List:

1. Edema in right UE
2. Decreased strength right UE and LE
3. Impaired balance
4. Impaired bed mobility
5. Impaired transfers
6. Nonfunctional gait
7. Decreased endurance

STGs (to be met in 1 to 2 weeks):

1. The patient will verbalize and demonstrate understanding of importance of right UE awareness, positioning, and protection.
2. Increase strength throughout the right hemibody by ½ grade each muscle group to allow for improved transfers, gait, and balance.
3. The patient will require minimal assistance for all bed mobility.
4. The patient will require moderate assistance consistently for all transfers via stand pivot from varying surfaces and going both left and right.
5. The patient will ambulate 50' with appropriate assistive device with moderate assistance.
6. The patient will require supervision for static sitting, moderate assistance for static standing, moderate assistance for dynamic sitting, and maximal assistance for dynamic standing.
7. Will improve endurance so that she is able to tolerate 1.5 to 2 hours of physical therapy daily for duration of stay.
8. Assess for need for right AFO.

LTGs (to be met in 3 to 4 weeks):

1. The patient will be independent with right UE management, care, and positioning.
2. The patient will increase right UE and LE strength by at least 1 grade so that functional mobility can be performed with supervision only.
3. The patient will be modified independent for all bed mobility.
4. The patient will require supervision for all transfers.

5. The patient will ambulate 150′ with appropriate assistive device with supervision and the appropriate bracing needs if necessary.
6. The patient will be independent with static sitting balance, modified independent for dynamic sitting balance, modified independent for static standing, and supervision for dynamic standing balance.
7. Recommend and obtain and educate on appropriate bracing as deemed necessary for improved function and safety.

P: The patient will be seen bid for 1.5 to 2 hours of physical therapy a day throughout duration of stay for neuromuscular re-education, strength, balance, and endurance training as well as functional mobility training with emphasis on goal attainment and the ability for the patient to discharge to home and care for herself and her child.

Mary Jane, PT

Note 1

One week later, you are working with the above 42 y.o. who suffered a left CVA with right hemiparesis. Today, the case manager comes to you and informs you that an insurance update is needed and that the insurance is starting to question the need for continued inpatient acute rehabilitation. She wants a copy of your note for today's session. Review the initial evaluation note so that you are able to make the appropriate comparison to today's treatment for justification of continued need for skilled physical therapy services and acute rehabilitation. Try to summarize how the patient is progressing toward her goals as established by the PT and write an appropriate plan that is consistent and within the above-stated plan of care.

Today the patient expresses her excitement and pleasure at the rate at which she is progressing and has high hopes of returning home soon. Today the patient required minimal assistance for all bed mobility and demonstrated the ability to incorporate the right UE into all tasks without the need for verbal reminders. Repetitive sit to stand and repetitive mat to w/c transfers via stand pivot performed for functional strength and endurance training with minimal assistance and only blocking of right knee 50% of the time secondary to fatigue. The patient ambulated 75′ x 1 and 50′ x 2 with LBQC with right ankle ace wrapped into DF with minimal assistance and manual assistance at the right LE for blocking and stabilization of the right knee during stance phase of gait to prevent buckling. The patient required rest breaks only between ambulation attempts for 1 to 2 minutes at a time. The patient continues to demonstrate right foot drop that likely requires a custom AFO. She also continues to demonstrate weakness in the right UE and LE evident by the need to manually block and stabilize the knee during transfers and gait as well as manual stabilization of the right UE secondary to weakness especially during the sit-to-stand transition.

Note 2

After 3 weeks in acute inpatient rehabilitation, the patient demonstrates readiness for discharge to home with assistance from her family. The family is apprehensive and is in the clinic today for family training. Please document in SOAP format the family training session and the patient's and family's response to the training and compare functional status findings from the previous note and initial evaluation. Also briefly comment on the status of her goals and write an appropriate plan. The patient performed all bed mobility at a modified independence level and is independent in the care and positioning of her right UE. All transfers performed with supervision and verbal cues for safety. The patient is able to don her right AFO with minimal assistance and ambulated 150′ with the LBQC with supervision. The family was educated on all functional mobility, proper guarding techniques, donning and doffing the AFO, as well as assessment of skin integrity and wearing instructions. The family demonstrated competence both verbally and physically with the ability to assist the patient in the home environment. The patient is slightly apprehensive about going home and expresses that she is still not independent with all functional mobility, which is where she would eventually like to be. She states that she would ultimately like to walk without an assistive device and no longer need the assistance from her family.

LOWER EXTREMITY AMPUTATION/ PROSTHETIC DEVICES

The following is an initial examination/evaluation for a patient recently admitted to an skilled nursing facility. Use it to help you complete the following 2 SOAP notes. Include the following in your notes:

- Write the A and P portions of the notes based on available information here and in the evaluative notes.
- Write your notes to maximize reimbursement.
- Be specific when documenting your interventions (patient education, coordination or communication with other disciplines, and procedural intervention).
- Write your A and P based on the plan of care provided and the patient's current status.

Date: January 15, 2011

Pr: 72-year-old male 4 days s/p right BKA

S: *History:* Long history of chronic wounds on the right foot; recently developed osteomyelitis and gangrene and underwent short transtibial (below-knee) amputation. *C/C:* Phantom pain 7/10 from the left foot, poor mobility, and decreased endurance. *Living situation:* Pt. is retired Army sergeant. Lives alone in single-level house, with 2 steps at the entrance. Has never used an assistive device. Has been independent with all ADL and IADL prior to admission. *PMH:* NIDDM, COPD,

PVD, and HTN. Pt. is a nonsmoker and nondrinker, although smoked 1 pack per day for 30 years. Quit when he was 50 y.o. Has one son living about 2 hours away who can assist on the weekends. Reports being active around his house and performing all home maintenance and yard work. Reports being an avid fisherman and participating in outdoor activities. *Pt.'s Goals:* Return to independent, active life style, including driving. Wants to obtain a prosthetic device. Communication: Pt. communicates goals and needs without difficulty.

O: *AROM:* (B) UEs are WNL; left LE is WNL; right hip flexion 90°, extension 0°, abduction 40°, adduction 10°, knee flexion 90°, knee extension –10°. *PROM:* Right knee extension –5°. *Strength:* (B) UEs and left LE are 4/5 throughout; right LE not assessed 2° to acuity. *Sensation:* Left LE is intact to light touch, right residual limb demonstrates diminished light touch sensation around suture line. *Incision:* Horizontal incision line at distal aspect of the residual limb, no tension, complete closure, no drainage. *Pulses:* Popliteal artery 2+ bilaterally. *Residual limb length:* 3" from tibial tuberosity.

Edema:	Right	Left
Knee joint	22 cm	20 cm
2" below	22.5 cm	19 cm
4" below	23 cm	18.5 cm

Balance: Not impaired when standing in parallel bars. Impaired while standing without UE support.
Bed Mobility: Independent rolling and scooting.
Transfers: Supine to and from sit with minimal assist x 1; sit to and from stand with minimal assist x 1; toilet transfers performed with minimal assist x 1.
Gait: Ambulated 10' x 1 in parallel bars with contact guard assist x 1 and 25' with standard walker with minimal assist x 1. Balance impaired when ambulating with walker 2° to decreased weight of right limb.
Wheelchair Management: Requires maximal assist for wheelchair parts management and can propel ~20' with verbal cues on level surfaces and then requires a rest break.
Endurance: Unable to ambulate more than 25' without shortness of breath.
Ther Ex: 20 minutes of exercises including hip AROM: Flexion, extension, abduction, and adduction; knee flexion and extension; hamstring stretching, and towel propping for the knee.

A: PT diagnosis: Impaired motor function, muscle performance, range of motion, gait, locomotion, and balance associated with amputation. Prognosis is good for anticipated goals and outcomes. Patient requiring skilled services for improving functional mobility including gait and transfer training with assistive devices due to amputation. Also required for preparing residual limb for prosthesis, improving joint mobility needed for prosthetic gait, education on skin integrity, gait training, and safe progression of mobility once he obtains the prosthetic device.

Problem List:
Impairments:
1. Decreased ROM right LE; especially hip extension and knee extension
2. Decreased strength right LE
3. Decreased sensation
4. Edema
5. Incision present
6. Impaired balance with walker
7. Phantom pain (7/10)
8. Decreased endurance

Activity Limitations/Participation Restrictions:
1. Decreased independence with ambulation
2. Decreased independence with transfers
3. Unable to perform home management tasks and care for his home
4. Unable to drive
5. Unable to perform necessary IADL (grocery shopping, going to bank, etc)
6. Unable to participate in usual active lifestyle

Anticipated Goals and Expected Outcomes:
After 8 to 12 weeks pt. will:
1. Demonstrate full A/PROM in the right LE with no contractures—necessary for normal prosthetic ambulation
2. Right LE strength 4/5 also to allow normal prosthetic ambulation
3. Be independent with skin care and monitoring skin with use of prosthesis
4. Demonstrate 100% healing of his incision
5. Report a 50% reduction in c/o phantom pain
6. Ambulate 500' with walker independently to allow home and limited community mobility
7. Ambulate 250' independently with prosthesis and least restrictive assistive device
8. Transfer in/out of bed independently and perform sit to and from stand independently
9. Participate in driving assessment to identify car modifications
10. Participate in a community outing with only minimal assist x1

P: See pt. for 1 hour bid for ~8 to 12 weeks to work on the above through active and passive exercise, endurance training, gait (including prosthetic) and transfer training, pain modulation to decrease phantom pain, balance, and patient education. The patient is motivated and agrees with the above plan.

Betty Bopp, PT

Note 1

The patient is now 2 weeks status post right transtibial amputation. He is continuing to complain of phantom pain (6/10) and sensation from the right foot. It resolves if he "squeezes" his residual limb. You are planning to attend a team conference for him on the following day,

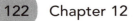

so you decide to take some objective measurements. Right AROM is as follows: hip flexion 120°, extension 5°, abduction 40°, adduction 10°, knee flexion 130°, knee extension –5°. PROM: Right knee extension 0°. Strength: Right LE hip flexion 4/5, extension holds against moderate resistance in side lying position, abduction holds against moderate resistance in side lying position; knee extension holds against minimal resistance in seated position; knee flexion holds against moderate resistance in side lying position. The patient cannot lie prone due to pulmonary problems and difficulty breathing when in this position. Skin: The incision is healing well. There is no drainage and no s/s of infection. It is moderately adhered to the underlying tissue and hypersensitive to pressure. Residual Limb Girth: 20 cm at the knee joint, 21 cm 2″ below, and 20 cm 4″ below. Function: The patient can move and transfer in and out of bed independently to a bedside commode or chair. He can manage the wheelchair parts with verbal cueing. He propels the wheelchair 50′ independently on level surfaces and carpet and then requires a rest. He can ambulate 75′ with a standard walker with supervision x 1 and good balance. You spent the next 15 minutes on patient education and exercise. You will discuss prosthetic options with the PT and if appropriate with the rehab team the following day.

Note 2

The patient is now 7 weeks s/p right transtibial amputation. He is continuing to complain of phantom pain (2/10) and sensation from the right foot occasionally, but it has decreased by about 75%. He has had a temporary prosthesis for about 2 days. Right AROM is as follows: hip flexion 120°, extension 10°, abduction 40°, adduction 10°, knee flexion 130°, knee extension 0°. Strength: Right LE hip flexion 4/5, extension holds against moderate resistance in side lying position, abduction holds against moderate resistance in side lying position; knee extension holds against moderate resistance in seated position; knee flexion holds against maximum resistance in side lying position. Skin: The incision is not adhered to the underlying tissue and sensitivity has subsided ~50%. Residual Limb Girth: 20 cm at the knee joint, 19 cm 2″ below, and 19 cm 4″ below. Function: He is independent with all wheelchair parts and transfer. He propels the wheelchair 500′ independently on level surfaces and carpet. He can ambulate 150′ with axillary crutches with supervision x 1 and good balance without the prosthesis. You spent 30 minutes on prosthetic training. He requires minimal assist to don and doff the socket. He ambulates 50′ with the prosthesis on and with axillary crutches with minimal assist for weight shifting. He is ambulating with an abducted gait on the prosthetic side. You spent 10 minutes educating the patient on skin precautions after removing the prosthesis and 15 minutes on exercises.

Musculoskeletal Trauma

The following is an initial examination/evaluation for a patient recently seen in an outpatient clinic. Use it to help you complete the following 2 SOAP notes. Include the following in your notes:

- Write the A and P portions of the notes based on available information here and in the evaluative notes.
- Write your notes to maximize reimbursement.
- Be specific when documenting your interventions (patient education, coordination or communication with other disciplines, and procedural intervention).
- Write your A and P based on the plan of care provided and the patient's current status.

Date: March 1, 2011

Referral from MD: 27 y.o. male s/p left wrist and ankle fracture; begin gentle wrist and ankle AROM & PROM; may begin using crutches with a platform for the left UE. PWB 50% on left lower extremity.

S: *HPI:* 4 weeks s/p fall (~25″) from a logging truck landing on his left side (2/1/11). Pt. sustained fracture of the left distal radius and ulna and left distal tibia and fibular. Pt. underwent ORIF for the wrist and ankle immediately after the injury. He was placed in a short-arm cast for the UE and short-leg cast for the LE. He was NWB on the left LE and has been unable to use crutches because he has not been allowed to bear weight on the affected UE. At the time of the fall, the pt. also sustained a mild concussion. He was hospitalized for 5 days following the injury. While hospitalized he received inpatient therapy to learn how to negotiate his wheelchair and perform transfers. Both casts were removed yesterday and his ankle was placed in a removable splint. Reports taking ibuprofen PRN for pain. *C/C:* Pain and stiffness in left UE & LE with decreased functional use of both. Doesn't like using wheelchair for mobility. Unable to work. Requiring assist with self-care activities and home management. *Living situation:* Right-hand dominant; lives with wife and 2 small children in single-level home with 2 steps @ entrance with a handrail on the right. Prior to injury the patient was employed by logging company and also worked as a contractor. He has been off work since the date of injury. Pt. is unable to drive and is relying on his wife & mother for transportation. No significant prior medical history or history of fracture. Reports being a nonsmoker and nondrinker. Family history is positive for OA. *Pt's Goals:* Return to previous level of function and RTW ASAP. Learn to ambulate with crutches.

O: *AROM:* Right UE & LE WNL; left shoulder, elbow, & hip WNL.

	AROM	PROM
Left wrist		
Flexion	20°	25°
Extension	10°	15°
UD	10°	15°
RD	15°	15°
Supination	30°	35°
Pronation	40°	45°
Left knee	0–100°	0–110°
Left ankle		
DF	-10°	-5
PF	20°	25°
Inversion	5°	5°
Eversion	0°	5°
Left hand: Pt. can perform a full fist but it is difficult 2° to edema, thumb IP, MCP, and CMC AROM is WNL		

Strength: Right UE & LE 5/5; left shoulder and hip 4/5; elbow, wrist, knee, & ankle deferred due to acuity.

Girth: Wrist figure 8 right: 36 cm left: 37.2 cm; ankle figure 8 right: 42 cm left: 44.1 cm.

Sensation: Left wrist and ankle intact to light touch & equal when compared to right.

Circulation: 2+ at radial & dorsal pedal arteries on the left Special Tests: N/A at this time due to acuity.

Gait: Unable to ambulate at this time. Transfers: Independent bed to and from chair, chair to and from toilet, sit to and from stand all NWB on left LE. Bed Mobility: Independent all areas.

DASH[3] Score: 78/100

Tx & HEP: AROM & PROM for left wrist for flexion, extension, & supination and for left ankle DF and PF, used opposite foot for self PROM of ankle; performed AROM for all digits and thumb; initiated compression glove for edema to be worn at night; instructed pt. in elevation and compression wrapping for ankle and wrist; instructed pt. in use of crutches with platform for left UE PWB 50% left using step to gait pattern. Pt. required contact guard assist x 1 for balance. The pt. performed all ex. independently and verbalized understanding of all precautions.

A: 27 y.o. RHD male 4 wks s/p fall. PT Diagnosis: Impaired mobility, muscle performance, and range of motion associated with fractures to the left wrist & ankle. Now with decreased AROM, PROM, and strength causing inability to ambulate, perform self-care or home management tasks without assistance, and inability to

work @ this time. Skilled services necessary to instruct patient in appropriate ther ex and progression, use of assistive device, & progression of gait as ordered. Pt. will also require strengthening and functional mobility retraining to prepare for return to normal living situation and RTW. Pt. able to communicate without limitations and demonstrates excellent motivation and good potential for full recovery. No comorbidities that could affect outcome identified at this time.

Anticipated Goals and Expected Outcomes:

At the end of 2 weeks, the pt. will:
1. Increase AROM 10–15° for the wrist, forearm, and ankle to allow normal functional activities
2. Decrease edema by 0.5 cm for the wrist and ankle to allow increased ROM
3. Ambulate with crutches with UE platform PWB left LE independently
4. Perform all self-care independently
5. Perform a full fist without limitations
6. DASH Score decreased 15%

At the end of 16 weeks (d/c), the pt. will:
1. Have AROM of the wrist, forearm, and ankle 90–100% of opposite to allow normal use during ADL, home management, and work activities
2. Grip and pinch strength will be 80–100% of right to allow normal use during ADL, home management, and work activities
3. Be independent with all self-care & home management tasks
4. Ambulate independently on all surfaces without the use of assistive device
5. Ascend and descend a flight of stairs independently without the use of an assistive device
6. Drive without restrictions
7. RTW at previous level of employment
8. DASH Score <20

P: See pt. 3x/wk for next 3–4 mos. to work on AROM & PROM of the wrist and ankle; general LE ex. for the hip, knee, shoulder, and elbow; gait training; functional mobility; & strengthening when appropriate. Will progress pt. as tolerated & according to MD orders. Pt. is in agreement with the above-stated plan.

John Smith, PT

Note 1

The patient is now 6 weeks s/p fall (has received 2 weeks of outpatient therapy). He is reporting improvement in his ability to perform self-care, achieve a full fist, and ambulate. He thinks the exercises are helping to improve all of these activities. He is seeing the doctor today and is hoping to be able to discontinue the use of the crutches. You take the following AROM measurements for the left wrist: flexion 50°, extension 35°, supination 50°, pronation 60°, left knee

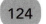

0–135°, left ankle –10° from neutral DF and has 45° of PF. He has 10° of inversion and 2° of eversion. He can perform all transfers independently and ambulates 100' independently PWB on the left LE with crutches with a left platform. Wrist figure 8 is 36.7 cm on the left and ankle figure 8 is 43.4 on the left. You are still not performing strength assessment due to fractures. You spend 45 minutes working on exercises to increase range of motion for the ankle and wrist and reviewing his home exercises.

Note 2

The patient is now 9 weeks s/p fall. He is reporting independence with self-care, ambulation, and driving. He thinks the exercises are helping to improve all of these activities and improve strength necessary for returning to work. He is ambulating full-weight-bearing on the left, without use of crutches. You take the following AROM measurements for the left wrist: flexion 80°, extension 65°, supination 75°, pronation 80°, left knee 0–140°, left ankle 0° (neutral) DF and has 50° of PF. He has 15° of inversion and 5° of eversion. He can ambulate for unlimited distances around the house and the community. He does have some mild swelling after ambulating distances greater than 400–500'. Wrist figure 8 is 36 cm on the left and ankle figure 8 is 43 on the left. Grip strength measured via grip dynamometer (#2 handle spacing) was 120 pounds on the right and 62 pounds on the left. You spend 45 minutes working on exercises to increase range of motion and for the ankle and wrist and reviewing his home exercises.

PEDIATRIC/ORTHOTIC DEVICES

The following is an initial examination/evaluation for a patient recently seen in an outpatient clinic. Use it to help you complete the following 2 SOAP notes. Include the following in your notes:

- Write the A and P portions of the notes based on available information here and in the evaluative notes.
- Write your notes to maximize reimbursement.
- Be specific when documenting your interventions (patient education, coordination or communication with other disciplines, and procedural intervention).
- Write your A and P based on the plan of care provided and the patient's current status.

Pr: 5-year-old female with L3 level myelomeningocele, referred to PT for transfer training, gait training, and KAFO management.

S: *Hx:* Myelomeningocele present at birth. Immediate surgery to repair. Resultant L3 incomplete paralysis. No history of hydrocephalus or seizure disorder. *C/C:* Impaired ability to transfer independently; decreased independence with ambulation. *L/S:* Lives with both parents, who are very supportive. Attends kinder-

garten at a local, public elementary school. *Pt.'s and parents' goals:* Increase independence with transfers, participate in circle time on the floor without having to be transferred by the teacher, ambulate household distances and short distances while at school independently, manage wheelchair independently. *Cognition/Communication:* Able to communicate without difficulty and expresses goals of therapy. At grade level for all school-related cognitive tasks per parental report.

O: *AROM:* Both UEs are WNL; LEs: hip flexion 120°, extension 0°, abduction 40°, adduction 10°, knee flexion 0°, knee extension 0°. *PROM:* Bilateral knees 0–135°; ankles DF 20° and PF 50°.

Strength: Both UEs 4/5 throughout; LEs: right hip flexion 3+/5, hip extension 3/5; abduction 3/5, adduction 3+/5; knee extension 3/5; left hip flexion 4/5, hip extension 3+/5; abduction 3+/5, adduction 4/5 knee extension 3+/5. All others are 0/5

Sensation: Left: Normal sensation in L1, 2, and 3 dermatomes; diminished in L4 and L5; absent in S1. Right: Normal sensation in L1 and 2; diminished in L3, L4, and L5; absent in S1.

Posture: Normal spinal alignment and absence of joint contractures or abnormal posture of feet and ankles.

Spasticity: Mild in both hip adductors, IR, and heel cords right > left. Modified Ashworth scale[2]: Right 2, Left 1+.

Bowel/Bladder: Incontinent in bowel and bladder control but is independently managed by parents and teacher.

Skin Condition: No impairments other than small area on right navicular from pressure from orthotic device.

Anthropometrics: Normal body weight for height.

Balance: Not impaired when standing in parallel bars with bilateral UE support.

Bed Mobility: Independent rolling and scooting.

Transfers: Supine to and from long and short sit independently; sit to and from stand with minimal assist x 1 using Lofstrand crutches and KAFOs; w/c to and from floor with max (A) x 1.

Floor Mobility: Independent in floor mobility for short distances using commando crawling.

Wheelchair Management/Mobility: Independent with mobility on level even surfaces for 50–60'; requires min (A) x 1 for managing parts including leg rests and arm rests.

Gait: Ambulated 10' x 1 with minimal assist x 1 using step to gait with KAFO knees locked at 0°. Balance impaired when ambulating with Lofstrands 2° to decreased proprioception and kinesthetic awareness of both LEs.

Endurance: Unable to ambulate more than 10' without shortness of breath.

Orthotic Devices: Dependent in donning and doffing.

A: PT Diagnosis: Impaired motor function and sensory integrity associated with nonprogressive disorder of the CNS. Prognosis for anticipated goals and outcomes is good. Skilled service needed to educate patient on appropriate ways to transfer and for endurance and strengthening to allow increased independence with gait and transfers.

Impairments:

1. Bilateral LE weakness
2. Flaccid ankles
3. Impaired proprioception and kinesthetic awareness during gait
4. Impaired sensation
5. Mild spasticity
6. Impaired endurance

Functional Limitations:

1. Decreased ability to transfer from wheelchair to floor
2. Decreased independence with sit to and from stand
3. Decreased independence with gait
4. Decreased ability to safely ambulate functional distances at home and at school
5. Requiring assistance for managing wheelchair parts
6. Requiring assist to manage orthotic devices

Anticipated goals and expected outcomes:

At the end of 8 weeks, the pt. will:

1. Transfer w/c to and from floor with minimal assist x 1
2. Perform sit to and from stand independently
3. Manage wheelchair leg rests and armrests independently
4. Propel w/c 500' independently
5. Ambulate 100' with KAFOs and bilateral Lofstrand crutches with close supervision
6. Don and doff the KAFOs with minimal assist

P: See pt. 2–3 x per week to work on the above plan and goals. Will require strengthening, endurance, balance, and gait training to meet above goals. Pt. and parent are in agreement with above plan.

Note 1

It is now the patient's fourth PT visit, and you have been working with this patient for the last 2 visits. She is very motivated and happy to come to therapy. She is very cooperative and her parents are very supportive and follow through with all instructions as assigned. She demonstrates the ability to transfer from the wheelchair to the floor with minimal assist and verbal cueing. She requires moderate assist to transfer from the floor to the wheelchair. Her UE strength is good via manual muscle test, but she cannot lift her own body weight at this point. She performs sit to and from stand with contact guard assist with the KAFOs and Lofstrand crutches. She can ambulate 40' with minimal assist of 1 with the braces and crutches also. Still demonstrating impaired dynamic balance. You worked with her for 30 minutes performing UE and LE strengthening and dynamic balance exercises and for an additional 15 minutes on gait training.

Note 2

The patient has been participating in PT for 1 month, you have seen her at every visit with the exceptions of the initial evaluation and during a re-evaluation that took place ~1–2 weeks ago. She is still very cooperative and motivated. She received new KAFOs from the orthotist today. They have a manual locking mechanism at the knee and are rigid at the ankles. Inspection of the devices reveals no problems with hardware and all edges and rivets are smooth and straps are well secured. The skin is free from breakdown before donning the devices. The patient requires moderate assist to don the orthotic devices and to engage the knee lock. She ambulated in the parallel bars 10' using an open-hand technique with minimal assist of one and then used her Lofstrands using a step to gait pattern also requiring minimal assist. After gait training (lasted ~20 minutes) the patient required moderate assist to doff the orthotic devices. Patient and parent were educated on skin inspection. There was a small area on the right navicular that was red after removing the device on the right. You provided education on monitoring the redness. Leaving the braces off, you performed 30 minutes of exercises for the UEs and LEs and dynamic balance activities.

References

1. Uniform Data System for Medical Rehabilitation. About the FIM system. Available at: http://www.udsmr.org/WebModules/FIM/FIM_About.aspx. Accessed January 28, 2012.
2. Bohannon Rw, Smith MB. Interrater reliability of a modified Ashworth scale of muscle spasticity. *Phys Ther.* 1987;67:206-207.
3. Hudak P, Amadio PC, Bombardier C, and the Upper Extremity Collaborative Group. Development of an upper extremity outcome measure: The DASH (Disabilities of the Arm, Shoulder, and Hand). *Amer J Ind Med.* 1996;29:602-608.

Glossary

abuse: Billing for items that are not covered or misusing billing codes. Usually a result of an error or lack of knowledge of proper code(s) or coding procedure(s).

activity limitation: Difficulties or limitations encountered by an individual who is attempting to complete a task or carry out an activity.

advance beneficiary notice (ABN): A notification that a health care provider asks a Medicare beneficiary to sign when providing a service that may not be covered by Medicare. In signing the ABN, the Medicare beneficiary agrees to pay for the service if it is not covered by Medicare.

assessment: The part of the SOAP note where the PT or PTA provides a summary outlining the patient's overall status or provides his or her impression of the patient.

carrier: A privately run insurance company that contracts with the government to pay bills for Medicare Part B. Carriers are determined by geographic region.

case-mix group: Categorization or grouping of patients in hospitals, or other facilities, according to common characteristics such diagnosis, disease, and functional status.

Centers for Medicare and Medicaid Services (CMS): A federal government agency that administers Medicare and works with state governments to administer Medicaid and State Children's Health Insurance Programs (SCHIP). CMS is housed within the Department of Health and Human Services (www.cms.hhs.gov).

comorbidity (or comorbidities): Aspect(s) of the patient's past medical history that affect(s) his or her current episode of care; a previous or current medical condition that has the potential to hinder progress in physical therapy.

copayment: The patient's responsibility for health care services provided; usually written in dollar amount and paid per visit; for example, $25 per physical therapy visit.

current procedural terminology: A coding system that is used for medical or health care procedures that is used within the health care delivery system.

deductible: The amount a patient must pay before insurance benefits begin; usually written in a dollar amount; for example, $1000 deductible.

diagnosis: A medical diagnosis assigned by a physician identifies the injury, illness, or disease, usually at the cellular, organ, or system level. A diagnosis assigned by a physical therapist identifies the impact of the patient's medical condition and impairments on movement and function.

diagnosis-related group (DRG): A categorization system used to group patients according to diagnosis, type of treatment, age, and other relevant criteria. DRGs are used as part of the inpatient prospective payment system.

disability: The inability or limitation in performing socially defined roles and tasks that would normally be expected of an individual within a given culture or environment.

disablement: The consequences of disease as they pertain to the relationship between body structures, the ability to carry out tasks, and the capability to function within society.

durable medical equipment (DME): Medical equipment that has been prescribed by a health care provider that is either purchased or rented by a patient, to be used

Erickson M, McKnight R. *Documentation Basics: A Guide for the Physical Therapist Assistant, Second Edition (pp. 127-130)*
© 2012 SLACK Incorporated

in the patient's home. Examples include hospital beds, walkers, canes, wheelchairs, and oxygen.

evaluation: An assessment of the patient's condition based on data collected during the physical therapist's examination. It includes consideration of the chronicity, severity, complexity, and extent of impairments, functional limitations, and disabilities.

evidence-based practice: Using the best evidence available (research reports, case studies, textbooks, etc), along with clinical experience, to make patient care decisions.

examination: A collection of tests and measurements, including questions to determine medical history, current complaints, lifestyle, and physical therapy goals. The examination data are used to identify pertinent physical therapy problems, comorbidities, and rehabilitation potential; to determine expected outcomes; and to develop a plan of care that includes appropriate interventions, consultation with other health care providers, and patient education.

fiscal intermediary (also known as *intermediary*): A privately run insurance company that contracts with the government to pay bills for Medicare Part A and some Medicare Part B. Fiscal intermediaries are determined by geographic region.

fraud: Billing an insurance company, Medicare, or other third-party payer for services that were not provided; billing for an item or service that has higher reimbursement than the service or item actually provided.

functional independence measure (FIM): A standardized multidisciplinary evaluation tool often used to score the patient's performance in self-care, bowel and bladder management, transfers, gait and/or wheelchair mobility, communication, and cognition. Patients are scored 1–7 (1 = *total assist* and 7 = *independent*) according to the level of assist he or she requires to complete the task.

functional limitation: An abnormality or limitation, caused by a pathology and/or impairment(s), that affects an individual's ability to carry out a meaningful action, task, or activity.

functional outcomes reporting (FOR): A type of medical record keeping that emphasizes patient function; the interventions and the patient's status are provided and organized according to the patient's functional problems.

health care clearinghouse: An entity associated with a health care provider or third-party payer that provides services such as billing, database management, transcription, information technology, etc. The health care clearinghouse has access to patient information but is not involved in patient care.

health maintenance organization (HMO): A type of third-party payment system or insurance company that only pays for health care provided within a given network.

home health care: Skilled nursing or rehabilitative care provided in a patient's home. Home care services can be provided when a patient is declared homebound.

homebound: Status given to a patient who is unable to leave his or her home or when leaving requires significantly taxing efforts. Short, infrequent trips, such as medical appointments and religious services, are permitted when a patient has been declared homebound.

impairment: A deviation or loss in a body function or structure.

incident report: A report filed in the event of an incident that could likely result in a lawsuit. Used to document errors and departures from normal procedures that result in adverse outcomes, procedural breakdowns, and catastrophic events. These reports are completed by the individual involved in the incident and are filed with the risk management department.

informed consent: Consent to a treatment(s) or service(s), provided by a patient after being informed of risks and benefits of treatment, alternatives to treatment, and consequences of no treatment at all.

inpatient rehabilitation facility (IRF): A hospital or unit within a larger facility (eg, acute care hospital) that provides intense rehabilitative services to patients. The majority of patients admitted to an IRF have been diagnosed with one of 13 qualifying medical conditions that have been established by Medicare. Examples are stroke, spinal cord injury, brain injury, amputation, hip fracture, burn, neurological disorder, and knee or hip replacement.

maintenance: Services that can be provided by a nonlicensed individual, including the patient himself, a family member, or a caregiver who has had some training from a skilled professional. Maintenance services are not reimbursed by Medicare or many other third-party payers.

malpractice: A bad or unskillful act performed by a physician or other professional provider that injures or causes harm to a patient or client; the failure of an individual or group to follow the accepted standards that have been set forth by their respective profession(s); includes willful negligence and ignorant malpractice.

managed care: A type of health care in which an insurance company (or third-party payer) maintains some control over costs and utilization of services and/or benefits.

Medicaid: A joint federal and state program that helps with medical costs for individuals with low incomes and limited resources.

medical necessity: As defined by Centers for Medicare & Medicaid Services, medical necessity is a procedure or intervention that is appropriate and needed for the diagnosis or treatment of a medical condition; is provided for the diagnosis, direct care, and treatment of a medical condition; meets the standards of good medical practice in the local area; and is not mainly for the convenience of the patient or health care provider.

Medicare physician fee schedule (MPFS): A list of procedures covered by Medicare and the amount reimbursed for each procedure

Medicare: The federal health insurance program for individuals: (1) 65 years of age and older who are receiving or eligible for social security retirement benefits; (2) younger than 65 with certain disabilities that meet the Social Security Act's disability requirements; and (3) with end-stage renal disease.

narrative: A type of medical record documentation where the information is provided in paragraph format.

objective: The portion of the SOAP note where the patient data are recorded; also includes treatment provided including patient education and/or collaboration/communication with other health care providers.

outcome: The end result of patient-client management. Could also be the end result of an episode of care.

participation restrictions: Problems an individual faces while involved in life situations.

pathology: Interruption or interference with the body's normal processes and simultaneous body efforts to heal itself or regain a normal state. Often known as the actual disease or medical diagnosis.

plan: The portion of the SOAP note where the PT or PTA describes plans for the upcoming session(s), discharge, patient education, collaboration with another provider, etc.

preferred provider organization (PPO): A type of third-party payment group or insurance company that includes a network of providers as well as out-of-network coverage available for the patient but at an increased cost compared to in-network providers.

primary care provider (PCP): A physician responsible for a patient's point of entry into the health care system. Some insurance companies require the PCP to be the patient's family physician. The PCP can also be a general practitioner, internal medicine specialist, or, in some cases, an obstetrician/gynecologist.

pro bono: A type of health care provided at no cost usually as a community service for individuals without health care benefits or means to pay for services.

problem-oriented medical record (POMR): A type of medical record keeping that organizes information and treatment according to patient problems.

prognosis: Includes the anticipated goals, expected frequency and duration of services, interventions to be used, expected outcomes, and ultimate plan for discharge.

prospective payment system (PPS): Medicare reimbursement provided to facilities (ie, hospitals and skilled nursing facilities) that is predetermined, or fixed, based on the patient's diagnosis and/or complexity.

protected health information (PHI): Individually identifiable information referring to an individual's medical history; previous, current, and future medical care; and billing and payment information. Also known as individually identifiable health information. Includes information that could potentially allow identification of the individual; for example, address, telephone and fax number, birth date, admission and discharge dates, voice recordings.

reimbursement: Payment made to a health care provider from an insurance company, or other third-party payer, after being billed for a service provided to a patient.

risk management: A way to minimize the possibility or risk of becoming involved in a lawsuit.

secondary insurance: Additional or supplemental insurance carried by a patient. Secondary insurance will typically cover additional costs not covered by the individual's primary insurance.

skilled care: A type of health care given when a patient needs management, observation, or evaluation by trained nurses or rehabilitation staff; also includes care that requires the unique judgment and skill of a trained individual for both safety and effectiveness.

skilled nursing facility (SNF): A freestanding facility, or facility within a hospital, nursing home, or rehabilitation center, that provides skilled medical, nursing, or rehabilitative services to patients. Examples of skilled services include intravenous injections, oxygen, feeding tubes, wound care, and rehabilitation.

state practice act: A state's regulation of licensed professionals. Usually defines the educational (and continuing education) requirements, scope of practice, acceptable service delivery, and licensure requirements.

subjective: A portion of the SOAP note where the PT or PTA records information provided by the patient, family member, and/or caregiver that is relevant to the episode of care.

template: A guide, checklist, standardized form, or list of items that should be included in documentation; followed to maintain consistency across patients and providers.

third-party payer: The insurance company, or other health benefit plan sponsor, that pays for medical services provided to a patient. The patient and the health care provider are considered the 2 primary parties.

utilization review: Examination of medical necessity, economic appropriateness, and quality of care provided to patients by a health care provider. Usually conducted by a managed care organization to determine the need for initiation or continuation of health care service.

Appendix A

Abbreviations and Symbols

This list provides many of the abbreviations and symbols used in medical charts and in physical therapy records. Because documentation styles can vary, you should check with your facility regarding abbreviations and symbols that are "approved" for use. Also, note that some abbreviations have more than one meaning. Be sure to understand the context in which each abbreviation is used. Lists are alphabetized by the abbreviation.

ABBREVIATIONS

A: or "A": assessment
a, (a), or (A): assist (min, mod, max)
AAROM: active assistive range of motion
Ab: antibody
abd: abduction
ABG(s): arterial blood gas(es)
ac: before meals
ACE: angiotensin-converting enzyme
Ach: acetylcholine
ACL: anterior cruciate ligament
ad lib: as desired
AD: assistive device; Alzheimer's disease
ADA: Americans with Disabilities Act
add: adduction
ADL: activities of daily living
ADM: abductor digiti minimi
AE: above elbow
AFB: acid-fast bacilli
AFO: ankle–foot orthosis
AGA: appropriate for gestational age
AIDS: acquired immunodeficiency syndrome

AK: above knee
AKA: above-knee amputation
ALL: acute lymphoblastic leukemia
ALS: amyotrophic lateral sclerosis
am: before noon
AMA: against medical advice
AMB or amb: ambulatory
AML: acute myeloblastic leukemia
ANOVA: analysis of variance
AP: ankle pump; anterior–posterior
APB: abductor pollicus brevis
APL: abductor pollicus longus
ARDS: adult (acute) respiratory distress syndrome
AROM: active range of motion
ASA: aspirin
ASAP: as soon as possible
ASHD: arteriosclerotic heart disease
ATF: anterior talofibular
AV: atriovenous
B, (B), bil: both or bilateral
BBB: blood–brain barrier
BE: below elbow
bid: twice daily
BK: below knee
BKA: below-knee amputation
BLE or (B)LE: bilateral lower extremities
BM: bowel movement
BMD: bone mineral density
BMI: body mass index
BP: blood pressure
BPH: benign prostatic hypertrophy
BPM or bpm: beats per minute
BRP: bathroom privileges

Erickson M, McKnight R. *Documentation Basics:*
A Guide for the Physical Therapist Assistant, Second Edition (pp. 131-136)
© 2012 SLACK Incorporated

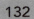

BSA: body surface area
BSC: bedside commode
BUN: blood urea nitrogen
C & S: culture and sensitivity
Ca: calcium
CA: cancer
CABG: coronary artery bypass graft
CAD: coronary artery disease
CAT: computerized axial tomography
CBC: complete blood count
c/c or C/C: chief complaint
cc or cm³: cubic centimeter
CCU: critical (or coronary) care unit
CDC: Centers for Disease Control
CF: calcaneofibular
CF: cystic fibrosis
CGA: contact guard assist
CHI: closed head injury
CHO: carbohydrate
Cl: chlorine
cm: centimeter
CMC: carpometacarpal
CMS: Center for Medicare & Medicaid Services
CMV: cytomegalovirus
CNS: central nervous system
c/o: complains of
COPD: chronic obstructive pulmonary disease
CORF: comprehensive outpatient rehabilitation facility
COTA: certified occupational therapist assistant
CP: cerebral palsy
CPAP: continuous positive airway pressure
CPM: continuous passive motion
CPR: cardiopulmonary resuscitation
CSF: cerebrospinal fluid
CT: computed tomography
CV: cardiovascular
CVA: cerebrovascular accident
CWP: cold whirlpool
cx: cancel; crutches
(D): dependent
DASH: Disabilities of the Arm, Shoulder and Hand disability questionnaire
DC: doctor of chiropractic; chiropractor
d/c: discharge or discontinue
DF: dorsiflexion
DI: dorsal interossei
DIP: distal interphalangeal
DJD: degenerative joint disease
DM: diabetes mellitus
DME: durable medical equipment
DMERC: durable medical equipment regional carrier
DO: doctor of osteopath
DOI: date of injury
DRG: diagnosis-related group
DRUJ: distal radioulnar joint

DTR: deep tendon reflex
DVT: deep vein thrombosis
dx: diagnosis
ea.: each
ECF: extracellular fluid
ECRB: extensor carpi radialis brevis
ECRL: extensor carpi radialis longus
ECU: extensor carpi ulnaris
EDC: extensor digitorum communis
EDM: extensor digiti minimi
EEG: electroencephalogram
EENT: eyes, ears, nose, and throat
EIP: extensor indicis proprius
EKG, ECG: electrocardiogram
EMG: electromyogram
EMS: emergency medical services
ENG: electronystagmograph
EO: elbow orthosis
EOB: edge of bed
EPB: extensor pollicus brevis
EPL: extensor pollicus longus
ERV: expiratory reserve volume
ESR: erythrocyte sedimentation rate
ESRD: end-stage renal disease
EtOH or ETOH: ethyl alcohol
ev, ever: eversion
ex.: exercise
F or 3/5: fair (manual muscle test)
FBS: fasting blood sugar
FCR: flexor carpi radialis
FCU: flexor carpi ulnaris
FDA: Food and Drug Administration
FDM: flexor digiti minimi
FDP: flexor digitorum profundus
FDS: flexor digitorum superficialis
FES: functional electrical stimulation
FEV: forced expiratory volume
FHR: fetal heart rate
fl: fluid
FM: fibromyalgia syndrome
FO: foot orthosis
FPB: flexor pollicus brevis
FPL: flexor pollicus longus
FRC: functional residual capacity
FTSG: full thickness skin graft
FUO: fever of unknown origin
FVC: forced vital capacity
FWB: full weight-bearing
FWW: front-wheeled walker
fx: fracture
G or 4/5: good (manual muscle test)
g: gram
GA: gestational age
GERD: gastroesophageal reflux disease
GH: glenohumeral

GI: gastrointestinal
GS: gluteal sets
GTT: glucose tolerance test
H & H: hemoglobin and hematocrit
H & P: history and physical
h or hr: hour
H_2O: water
HAV: hepatitis A virus; hallux abductovalgus
Hb: hemoglobin
HBV: hepatitis B virus
HCFA: Health Care Financing Administration
HCPCS: health care common procedure coding system
Hct: hematocrit
HCV: hepatitis C virus
HDL: high-density lipoprotein
HEP: home exercise program
HHA: home health agency
HIV: human immunodeficiency virus
HMO: health maintenance organization
HNP: herniated nucleus pulposus
h/o: history of
HO: hand orthosis
HO: hip orthosis
HOB: head of bed
HP: hot pack
HPI: history of present illness
HR: handrail; heart rate
HRT: hormone replacement therapy
HTN: hypertension
hx: history
Hz: hertz
(I): independent
I & D: incision and drainage
I & O: intake and output
IADL: instrumental activities of daily living
IC: inspiratory capacity
ICD: *International Classification of Diseases*
ICF: intracellular fluid; *International Classification of Functioning, Disability, and Health*
ICIDH: *International Classification of Impairments, Disabilities, and Handicaps*
ICP: intracranial pressure
ICU: intensive care unit
IDDM: insulin-dependent diabetes mellitus
IDEA: Individuals with Disabilities in Education Act
Ig: immunoglobulin
IM: intramuscular
INH: isoniazid
inv: inversion
IP: inpatient; interphalangeal
IPPS: inpatient prospective payment system
IRV: inspiratory reserve volume
IV: intravenous
K: potassium
KAFO: knee–ankle–foot orthosis
kg: kilogram

L: liter
L or (L): left
LAC: long-arm cast
LAQ: long arc quadriceps exercise
LB: lower body
LBQC: large-base quad cane
LCL: lateral collateral l=igament
LDL: low-density lipoprotein
LE: lower extremity
LHD: left-hand dominant
LLC: long-leg cast
LMN: lower motor neuron
LMRP: local medical review policies
LP: lumbar puncture
L/S, l/s: lifestyle
LT: lunotriquetrial
LTFG: long-term functional goal
LTG: long-term goal
LTM: long-term memory
m: meter
m.: muscle
MAS: Modified Ashworth Scale
max: maximum
MCA: motorcycle accident
MCL: medial collateral ligament
MCP: metacarpophalangeal
MD: muscular dystrophy; medical doctor/physician
MED(s): medicines, medications
MG: myasthenia gravis
MHP: moist hot pack
MHz: megahertz
MI: myocardial infarction
MID: multi-infarct dementia
min: minimal
mm: millimeter
mm Hg: millimeters of mercury
MMT: manual muscle test
mod: moderate
MOI: mechanism of injury
mos: months
MRI: magnetic resonance image
MRSA: methicillin-resistant *Staphylococcus aureus*
MS: multiple sclerosis
MTP: metatarsophalangeal
mV: millivolt
MVA: motor vehicle accident
N or 5/5: normal (manual muscle test)
N: Newton
n & v: nausea and vomiting
n.: nerve
Na: sodium
N/A: not applicable
n.s.: at bedtime
NBQC: narrow base quad cane
NDT: neurodevelopmental treatment
NICU: neonatal intensive care unit

NIDDM: non-insulin-dependent diabetes mellitus
NIH: National Institutes of Health
NMES: neuromuscular electrical stimulation
NPO: nothing by mouth
NSAID(s): nonsteroidal anti-inflammatory drug(s)
NT: not tested
NWB: non-weight-bearing
O: or "O": objective
O_2 or O2: oxygen
OA: osteoarthritis
OASIS: outcome & assessment information set
OB/GYN: obstetrics and gynecology
OBS: organic brain syndrome
OCD: obsessive–compulsive disorder
ODM: opponens digitit minimi
OI: osteogenesis imperfecta
OOB: out of bed
OP: opponens pollicus; outpatient
OR: operating room
ORIF: open reduction internal fixation
OSHA: Occupational Safety & Health Administration
OT: occupational therapist
OTC: over-the-counter (ie, drugs)
OTR/L: occupational therapist registered and licensed
oz: ounce
P or 2/5: poor (manual muscle test)
p: probability of success
p!: pain
P: or "P": plan
PA: posterior–anterior
PA-C: physician assistant
pc: after meals
PCA: patient-controlled anesthesia
PCL: posterior cruciate ligament
PD: Parkinson's disease
PDR: *Physicians' Desk Reference*
PE: pulmonary embolism
PEG: percutaneous endoscopic gastrostomy (tube)
PERRLA: pupils equal, round (regular), reactive to light, and accommodating
PET: positron emission tomography
PF: plantarflexion
PFT: pulmonary function test
PI: palmar interossei
PIP: proximal interphalangeal
PL: palmaris longus
PLOF: prior level of function
pm: after noon
PMH: past (or previous) medical history
PNF: proprioceptive neuromuscular facilitation
PNS: peripheral nervous system
po: by mouth
POMR: problem-oriented medical record
post-op: postoperative
PPO: preferred provider organization
PPS: prospective payment system

PQ: pronator quadratus
PRN: as needed
PROM: passive range of motion
PRUJ: proximal radioulnar joint
PT: physical therapist; pronator teres; prothrombin time
Pt. or pt.: patient
PTA: physical therapist assistant; prior to admission
PTCA: percutaneous transluminal coronary angioplasty
PTF: posterior talofibular
PTT: partial thromboplastin time
PVD: peripheral vascular disease
PWB: partial weight-bearing (usually 50% unless otherwise indicated; may need to check with physician to clarify)
q: every
q2h: every 2 hours
q3h: every 3 hours
q4h: every 4 hours
q8h: every 8 hours
qam: every morning
qh: every hour
qid: 4 times a day
qod: every other day
QS: quad set/quadriceps set
R or (R): right
RA: rheumatoid arthritis
RBC: red blood cell
RC: radiocarpal
RCL: radial collateral ligament
RD: radial deviation
RDS: respiratory distress syndrome
reps: repetitions
RGO: reciprocating gait orthosis
RHD: right-hand dominant
r/o; R/O: rule out
ROM: range of motion
ROS: review of systems
RPE: rate of perceived exertion
RR: respiratory rate
r/s: reschedule
RT: respiratory therapy
RTC: return to clinic
RTW: return to work
RV: residual volume
Rx: prescription
s or SVN: supervision
S: or "S": subjective
SAC: short-arm cast
SaO_2: oxygen saturation
SAQ: short arc quadriceps exercise
SBA: standby assist
SCI: spinal cord injury
SIDS: sudden infant death syndrome
SL: scapholunate; side lying
SLC: short-leg cast
SLE: systemic lupus erythematosus

SLP: speech language pathologist
SLR: straight-leg raise
SMA: spinal muscular atrophy
SO: shoulder orthosis
SOB: shortness of breath
s/p: status post
SPT: student physical therapist
SPTA: student physical therapist assistant
s/s: signs and/or symptoms
ST: scapulothoracic
stat: immediately
STG: short-term goal
STM: short-term memory
STSG: split-thickness skin graft
T or 1/5: trace (manual muscle test)
T: temperature
TA: therapeutic activity
TB: tuberculosis
TBI: traumatic brain injury
tbsp or T: tablespoon
TFCC: triangular fibrocartilagenous complex
THA: total hip arthroplasty
THR: total hip replacement
TIA: transient ischemic attack
tid: 3 times a day
TKA: total knee arthroplasy
TKE: terminal knee extension
TKR: total knee replacement
TMJ: temporomandibular joint
TP: therapeutic procedure
TPN: total parenteral nutrition
tsp or t: teaspoon
TTP: tender to palpation
TTWB: toe-touch weight-bearing
TV: tidal volume
tx: traction or treatment
UCL: ulnar collateral ligament
UD: ulnar deviation
UE: upper extremity
UMN: upper motor neuron
US: ultrasound
UTI: urinary tract infection
UV: ultraviolet
V: volt
v/c: verbal cue(s)
W: watt
WBAT: weight bearing as tolerated
WBC: white blood cell
WBQC: wide-base quad cane

w/c: wheelchair
w/cm^2: watts per centimeters squared
WFL: within functional limits
WHFO: wrist–hand–finger orthosis
WHO: wrist–hand orthosis; World Health Organization
wk: week
WNL: within normal limits
WP: whirlpool
WWP: warm whirlpool
y.o.: year old

COMMON SYMBOLS

about: ~
after: $\bar{p}$
ascend or increase: ↑
at: @
before: $\bar{a}$
degrees Celsius: °C
degrees Fahrenheit: °F
degrees: °
descend or decrease: ↓
equal, equal to: (=)
extension: /
female: ♀
flexion: : ✓
greater than, greater than or equal to: >, ≥
hour, foot: '
inch, minute: "
less than, less than or equal to: <, ≤
male: ♂
micrometer: µ
negative: (–) or –
not equal to, unequal: ≠
number of individuals assisting (one, two): x1, x2
parallel (as in parallel bars): // (// bars)
per: /
positive: (+) or +
possible, question, suggestive: ?
pounds: # or lbs.
primary: 1°
sample mean: $\bar{x}$
secondary, secondary to: 2°, 2° to
times (as in 3 times per day): x (3x/day)
to/from: ↔
up and down or ascend and descend: ↑↓
with: $\bar{c}$
without: $\bar{s}$

Appendix B

Sample Forms and Templates

Jeff Erickson, PT, MS, SCS, ATC, CSCS

Erickson M, McKnight R. *Documentation Basics:*
A Guide for the Physical Therapist Assistant, Second Edition (pp. 137-150)
© 2012 SLACK Incorporated

GENERAL PHYSICAL THERAPY EVALUATION FORM

Note: These forms are not labeled S, O, A, P but generally follow the SOAP format.

Patient's Name _____   Age: _____   Date: _____

Physician: _____   Diagnosis: _____

Reason for Referral _____

Injured Side: ❑ Right   ❑ Left   Hand Dominance: ❑ Right   ❑ Left

History

HPI: _____

_____

_____

History of Similar Problem: ❑ No   ❑ Yes _____

C/C: _____

Pain Scale (0–10): _____

Activities That Increase Pain: _____

Activities That Decrease Pain: _____

Previous Treatment: _____

Diagnostic Testing/Imaging _____

Numbness/Tingling: ❑ No   ❑ Yes _____

Temperature Changes: ❑ No   ❑ Yes _____

Orthotic/Prosthetic Devices: ❑ No   ❑ Yes _____

Living Situation

Lives With_____

Home Environment: _____

Employment/Work/School Status:_____

Occupation: _____

PMH:_____

Family Medical History: _____

Current Medication(s): _____

Social/Health Habits (Smoking/Drinking Alcohol): _____

Functional Status: _____

ADLs: _____

IADLs:_____

Patient's Goals: _____

Gross Review of Systems

Cardiovascular System: HR _____   RR _____   BP _____

Integumentary System: ❏ Not Impaired   ❏ Impaired_____

_____

Neuromuscular System: ❏ Not Impaired   ❏ Impaired_____

_____

Musculoskeletal System: ❏ Not Impaired   ❏ Impaired_____

_____

Communication/Affect/Cognition: ❏ Not Impaired   ❏ Impaired_____

_____

Tests and Measurements

Aerobic Capacity/Endurance: _____

Girth/Other Anthropometric Assessment:
Landmark   Right   Left

_____   _____   _____
_____   _____   _____
_____   _____   _____

Circulation:
Pulse(s)   Right   Left

_____   _____   _____
_____   _____   _____

Cranial/Peripheral Nerve Integrity:
Test:_____   Results: _____

_____

Test:_____   Results: _____

_____

Test:_____   Results: _____

_____

Functional Assessment:
_____

_____

Gait/Locomotion/Balance:
Gait: _____
Transfers:_____
Bed Mobility: _____
Balance Assessment: _____
Other Functional Mobility: _____
Other Functional Mobility: _____
Other Functional Mobility: _____

Integumentary Condition:
Type of Wound: _____
Location: _____
Appearance: _____
Size:_____   Odor: _____
Drainage:_____
Tunneling: _____   Periwound Area:_____
See attached sketch.

ROM:

AROM   Joint: Right   Left

_____   _____   _____
_____   _____   _____
_____   _____   _____
_____   _____   _____

PROM   Joint: Right   Left

_____   _____   _____
_____   _____   _____
_____   _____   _____
_____   _____   _____
_____   _____   _____

Strength: Joint: Right   Left

_____   _____   _____
_____   _____   _____
_____   _____   _____
_____   _____   _____
_____   _____   _____

Posture: _____
_____

Flexibility   Joint: Right   Left

_____   _____   _____
_____   _____   _____
_____   _____   _____
_____   _____   _____

Reflexes   Reflex: Right   Left

_____   _____   _____
_____   _____   _____
_____   _____   _____
_____   _____   _____

Special Tests   Test: Right   Left

_____   _____   _____
_____   _____   _____
_____   _____   _____
_____   _____   _____
_____   _____   _____

Intervention(s) (Including patient education and HEP): _____
_____
_____
_____

Total Treatment Time: _____

Assessment and Plan

Summary: _____

Physical Therapy Diagnosis: _____

Skilled Services Needed for: _____

Impairments/Functional Problems

      _____   _____   _____

      _____   _____   _____

      _____   _____   _____

Barriers to Rehab/Comorbidities/Complexities: _____

Prognosis: _____

Potential for Rehabilitation: _____

Expected Outcomes (LTGs): _____
_____
_____
_____

Plan (Including description and rationale of interventions, expected frequency and duration of services, ultimate plan for discharge): _____
_____
_____
_____

Therapist's Signature _____
Date_____

KNEE EVALUATION FORM

Patient's Name _____   Age: _____   Sex: _____   Date: _____
Sport(s)/Occupation:_____   School/Employer: _____
Physician Hx: _____   Next Dr. Visit: _____
Dx/Surgical Procedure: _____   Date of Surgery: _____
Treatment Requested/Special Precautions: _____

Subjective:

Injured Knee: ❏ Right   ❏ Left   Dominant Leg: ❏ Right   ❏ Left
Onset: ❏ Acute   ❏ Chronic   Date of Injury: _____
History/Mechanism: _____
_____
_____

Previous Injury: ❏ Yes   ❏ No   Similar Injury: ❏ Yes   ❏ No
Prior Treatment: _____
Chief Complaint: _____
ADL Limitations: ❏ Stairs   ❏ Uneven Ground   ❏ Squatting   ❏ Driving
                       ❏ Walking   ❏ Work/Household/Recreation Activities
                       ❏ Other_____
X-rays/MRI:_____
Pain Rating (0–10): _____   Rest:_____   Activity:_____
Location: _____
Better: _____   Worse: _____
Numbness/Tingling? ❏ Yes   ❏ No   Where: _____
Global Rating (0–100): _____
Does Knee?   Catch/Pop (Y/N)   Give Way (Y/N)   Swell (Y/N)   Sublux/Dislocate (Y/N)
Orthotics/Sleeves:_____   Injections (Y/N) # _____   Last:_____
PMH/Prior Surgeries: _____
Meds:_____
Hobbies/Activities/Work Duties: _____
Pt. Goals:_____
Other: _____

Objective

General Observations: _____
Discoloration: ❏ Yes   ❏ No   Where: _____
Swelling/Effusion: ❏ None   ❏ Minimal (1+)   ❏ Moderate (2+)   ❏ Severe (3+)
      Where: _____
Skin Temperature (Circle):   Normal   Warm   Cold
Patellar Position/Tracking: _____   Patellar Mobility (↑, N, ↓): Sup ___   Inf ____   Lat ____   Med____
AROM: ❏ Right ❏ Left   PROM: ❏ Right ❏ Left   Strength: ❏ Right ❏ Left
Hip Flexion _____
Knee ROM _____
Ankle DF/PF _____
Ankle IV/EV _____
Gait: _____
Assistive Device: ❏ None   ❏ Crutches   ❏ Cane   ❏ Walker   ❏ Other:_____
Weight Bearing Status: NWB   PWB (_____%)   FWB
Palpation: _____

Girth Measurements: Right   Left   Units (Circle): cm in

_____ Below   _____   _____

_____ MJL   _____   _____

_____ Above   _____   _____

_____ Above   _____   _____

_____ Above   _____   _____

Functional Strength: Right   Left

 Quad Set   _____   _____

 Flexion SLR   _____   _____

 Extensor Lag ❏ Yes (___°) ❏ No ❏ Yes (___°) ❏ No

Special Tests:

Ant. Drawer:	L _____	R_____	Post. Drawer:	L _____	R _____
Lachman's:	L _____	R_____	Pivot Shift:	L _____	R _____
Valgus (0°):	L _____	R_____	Valgus (30°):	L _____	R _____
Varus (0°):	L _____	R_____	Varus (30°):	L _____	R _____
McMurray (IR):	L _____	R_____	McMurray (ER):	L _____	R _____
Apprehension:	L _____	R_____	Apley Compr:	L _____	R _____
Post. Sag:	L _____	R_____	Noble Compr:	L _____	R _____

 Other: _____

Flexibility:

Prone Quad:	L _____	R_____	ITB:	L _____	R _____
Hams:	L _____	R_____	Gastrocs:	L _____	R _____
Thomas Hip					
Flexor:	L _____	R_____			

 Other: _____

Neurovascular Tests: Sensation: _____ Capillary Refill: L _____ R _____

 Patellar Reflex: L _____ R_____ Achilles Reflex: L _____ R _____

Biomechanical Screen: _____

Leg Length: L _____ R_____ Short Leg: L _____ R_____ Symmetrical ___

Single Leg Stance (eyes open/closed): L _____ seconds R _____ seconds

 Other: _____

Other Objective Tests/Measurements _____

_____

_____

_____

_____

Treatment: _____ Ice   _____ E-Stim _____ US/Phono _____ Russian

    _____ Biofeedback (__uV) _____ Whirlpool (Cold/Warm/Contrast)

    _____ Ionto (Dex Lidocaine) Other: _____

#1 Parameters:_____ Time: _____minutes

#2 Parameters:_____ Time: _____minutes

Other (Pat. Mobs/Stretching): _____

HEP Instruction and Performance (Time: ____ minutes):

_____ Quad Sets	_____ Glute Sets	_____ Heel Slides	_____ Seated Flexion
_____ HC Stretch	_____ HS Stretch	_____ Quad Stretch	_____ Hip Flex Stretch
_____ ITB Stretch	_____ Pat. Mobs	_____ Heel Props	_____ Mini-Squats
_____ Wall Squats	_____ Heel Raises	_____ Nose Touches	_____ Step-Ups
_____ SLR's (F, E, Abd, Add)		_____ Tubing SLR's (F, E, Abd, Add)	

Other: _____

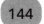

EVALUATION/PLAN OF CARE

PT Diagnosis: _____

_____

Need for skilled care:

Problems List:
Impairments: *Activity Limitations and Participation Restrictions*:

❏ Pain   ❏ Decreased Patellar Mobility   ❏ Gait/Stair Mobility
❏ Decreased ROM   ❏ Decreased LE Flexibility   ❏ Uneven Terrain
❏ Decreased Strength   ❏ Poor LE Biomechanics   ❏ Squatting
❏ Swelling/Effusion   ❏ Decreased Balance   ❏ Work/Recreation IADL
❏ Dependence With HEP   ❏ Driving
Other: _____   Other: _____

Short-Term Goals (Time Frame _____ Weeks/Visits):

_____
_____
_____
_____
_____

Long-Term Goals (Time Frame _____ Weeks/Visits):

_____
_____
_____
_____
_____

Safety Precautions/Risk Factors/Barriers to D/C: _____

_____

Rehab Potential/Prognosis: ❏ Good   ❏ Fair   ❏ Poor
Treatment:_____
Frequency:_____ Duration: _____

Therapist: _____ Date: _____

Physical Therapy Assessment and Plan of Care*

Patient Name: _____   Patient's DOB: _____   PT Examination Date: _____

** For the physician:
I have read and concur with the plan of care written below for this patient:

_____   _____   _____

Name of Supervising Physician   **Physician Signature**   **Date**

Summary/Comments: _____

_____

_____

Primary Medical Diagnosis: _____   (ICD-9): _____

PT Diagnosis (relates impairments to function): _____

Comorbidities Influencing Treatment (and ICD-9): _____

Patient's Rehab Potential: _____

Skilled Services Required for: _____

Problem List:

Physical therapy impairments:

1. _____
2. _____
3. _____
4. _____
5. _____

Activity Limitations/Participation Restrictions
(Include ADL, home management, community, work, leisure):

1. _____
2. _____
3. _____
4. _____
5. _____

Expected Outcomes (to be met by_____):

A. _____
B. _____
C. _____
D. _____
E. _____

STGs (to be met by_____):

A-1. _____
B-1. _____
C-1. _____
D-1. _____
E-1. _____

Treatment Plan

Frequency/Duration Services Will Be Provided: _____

Physical therapy modality/procedure codes:

1. _____   4. _____
2. _____   5. _____
3. _____   6. _____

❏ The patient/care giver is in agreement with the plan.

Examination, assessment, and plan of care completed and written by:

_____

(PT Signature)

*Reprinted with permission from Erickson ML, McKnight R, Utzman RR. *Physical Therapy Documentation: From Examination to Outcome.* Thorofare, NJ: SLACK Incorporated; 2008.

SAMPLE PROGRESS REPORT*

Patient Name: _____ Dates of Service: _____

Date Progress Report Written _____

Subjective Report:_____
_____
_____
_____
_____
_____
_____

Objective Measurements:_____
_____
_____
_____
_____
_____
_____

Current Outcome Goals to Be Met By _____

Progress Toward Goals:
A._____
B. _____
C._____
D._____
E. _____
F. _____

Changes to Plan of Care and Rationale: _____
_____
_____
_____
_____
_____

Plans for Further Interventions: _____
_____
_____
_____
_____
_____

*Reprinted with permission from Erickson ML, McKnight R, Utzman RR. *Physical Therapy Documentation: From Examination to Outcome.* Thorofare, NJ: SLACK Incorporated; 2008.

PHYSICAL THERAPY ASSESSMENT AND PLAN OF CARE

Patient's Name: John Woods   Age: 16   Date: 2/11/2012
Physician: Self-referred   DOB: 1/12/1996   Diagnosis: Right ankle sprain
Medical Record Number: 000102301

Problem

Rec'd call from patient's mother stating that pt. sprained his ankle at a basketball game on 02/10/2012.

History

HPI: 16 y.o. male who plays basketball. Last night sustained an injury via PF and inversion mechanism after landing on another player's foot. Reports that he fell and felt a pop. Reports sudden pain and inability to move or weight bear on the right LE

History of Similar Problem: ☐ No   ☑ Yes: Patient treated here 6 months ago for left ankle sprain
C/C: Pain, stiffness, swelling, discoloration, inability to walk or weight bear on the right LE
Pain Scale (0–10): 6/10
Activities That Increase Pain: weight bearing, inversion, and DF
Activities That Decrease Pain: ice, rest, elevation
Previous Treatment: ice, rest, elevation
Diagnostic Testing/Imaging: none at this point
Numbness/Tingling: ☑ No   ☐ Yes _____
Temperature Changes: ☐ No   ☑ Yes: Reports warmth around the ankle joint
Orthotic/Prosthetic Devices: ☐ No   ☑ Yes: Using an Ace wrap that was applied by the athletic trainer after the injury

Living Situation

Lives With: Parents and younger sibling
Home Environment: Has a flight of stairs to get to his bedroom and 2 steps at the entrance
Employment/Work/School Status: Pt. is a high school junior who participates regularly in sports including basketball, soccer, and baseball
Occupation: N/A
PMH: left ankle sprain 7/1/11, left knee ACL reconstruction 5/30/2010
Family Medical History: (+) OA; HTN
Current Medication(s): OTC anti-inflammatory medication
Social/Health Habits (Smoking/Drinking Alcohol): Non-drinker, non-smoker
Functional Status: Unable to walk without limp, can't ambulate around school; can't participate in recreational activities
    ADLs: Limited due to inability to bear weight on the right leg
    IADLs: Unable to ambulate in the community
Patient's Goals: Decrease pain and swelling; return to normal walking; return to recreational activity

Gross Review of Systems

Cardiovascular System: HR:77 bpm   RR:12 resp/min   BP:120/86
Integumentary System: ☑Not impaired   ☐Impaired
Neuromuscular System: ☑Not impaired   ☐Impaired
Musculoskeletal System: ☐Not impaired   ☑Impaired—decreased ROM right ankle—see below
Communication/Affect/Cognition: ☑Not impaired   ☐Impaired

Tests and Measurements

Observation: Gross joint effusion; ecchymosis in the ankle joint, dorsum of the foot and around the calcaneal area

Palpation: Point tender over the lateral calcaneofibular ligaments; No point tenderness over any bony structures

Girth/Other Anthropometric Assessment:

Landmark	Right	Left
Ankle Figure 8	53.8 cm	51 cm
Bimalleolar	28 cm	26 cm

Circulation:

Pulse(s)	Right	Left
Dorsalis pedis	2+	2+

Cranial/Peripheral Nerve Integrity:

Test: Light touch   Results: Intact to light touch; equal bilateral

Self-report questionnaire: Lower Extremity Functional Scale = 20

Gait/Locomotion/Balance: Gait: Ambulated into the clinic without assistive device; decreased weight bearing and stance time on the right due to pain; decreased stride length. After instruction pt. was able to ambulate with bilateral axillary crutches WBAT on (R) LE unlimited distance using step to gait pattern.

Transfers: Independent

Bed Mobility: Independent

Balance Assessment: Not assessed due to pain and injury acuity

ROM:

AROM	Joint:	Right	Left
	Ankle DF	-5°	8°
	Ankle PF	15°	50°

Strength:

	Joint:	Right	Left
	Ankle DF	Not tested	5/5

Posture: Ankle positioned in slight PF

Flexibility: Not assessed due to pain

Special Tests:

Test:	Right	Left
Anterior drawer	(+2)	(-)
Talar tilt test	(+2)	(-)
Tap test	(-)	(-)
Metatarsal compression	(-)	(-)
Tib fib compression	(-)	(-)

Intervention(s) (Including patient education and HEP):

Ice and interferential electrical stimulation to the right ankle 100-150Hz x 20 minutes with elevation. Exercises and HEP Rx included: ankle pumps x5'; heel cord stretch 15 seconds x 10 reps; hip SLR x4 3 sets 15; ace wrap applied for compression; instruction in crutches as above. Total Treatment Time: 60'

Assessment

Summary and PT diagnosis: 16 y.o. male 1 day s/p Grade II ankle sprain with pain, swelling, and limited ROM and weight bearing limiting ability to ambulate without assistive device; unable to walk around school environment or participate in recreational activities.

Skilled services needed for: administering modalities to decrease pain and swelling, safely restoring ROM, gradually progressing back to normal weight bearing. Will also require implementation of safe functional drills prior to return to activity for safety

Impairments	*Activity limitations/Participation restrictions*
Pain	Impaired mobility including any weight bearing activities
Swelling	Unable to participate in mobility to change classes at school
Decreased AROM	Unable to perform normal recreational activities
Associated weakness	

Barriers to Rehab/Co-morbidities/Complexities: None

Prognosis:

Potential for Rehabilitation: Excellent potential to meet goals stated below

Expected Outcomes (Long-term goals) To be met in 4-6 weeks:

1. Decrease pain from 6/10 to 0-1/10
2. Normalize girth to equal the left side
3. Restore 100% of the AROM on the left
4. Increase Lower Extremity Functional Scale score to > 72.
5. Pain free weight bearing during walking and running tasks
6. Full weight bearing gait without pain for unlimited distances at school and in the community
7. Full return to recreational activity without limitation

Plan

(Including description and rationale of interventions, expected frequency and duration of services, ultimate plan for discharge):

See the pt. 2-3x/week for 4-6 weeks to work on the above impairments and functional deficits. He will require modalities to decrease pain and swelling, ther ex to restore ROM and strength, instruction in elevation and compression to control edema, gait training, weaning from assistive device as weight bearing improves, and functional drills to allow pt. to safely return to full school and recreational participation. If there is no improvement in weight bearing or point tenderness will call patient's primary care provider and make referral for radiograph.

☑ The plan of care described above has been reviewed with the patient/parent. They are in agreement.

_____

Therapist's signature   Date

References

1. American Physical Therapy Association. *Guide to Physical Therapist Practice.* Alexandria, Va: American Physical Therapy Association; 2001. Available at: guidetoptpractice.apta.org. Accessed February 18, 2012.

2. Centers for Medicare and Medicaid Services. Pub. No. 100-02 Medicare Benefit Policy Manual, Chapter 15-Section 220. Available at: http://www.cms.gov/Manuals/IOM/ItemDetail.asp?ItemID=CMS012673. Published 2006. Accessed February 3, 2012.

3. Erickson ML, McKnight R, Utzman RR. *Physical Therapy Documentation: From Examination to Outcome.* Thorofare, NJ: SLACK Incorporated; 2008.

4. American Physical Therapy Association. Documentation templates. In: *Guide to Physical Therapist Practice.* Alexandria, Va: American Physical Therapy Association; 2001. Available at: guidetoptpractice.apta.org. Accessed February 18, 2012.

5. American Physical Therapy Association. Defensible documentation for patient/client management. Available at: http://www.apta.org/Documentation/DefensibleDocumentation. Accessed February 1, 2012.

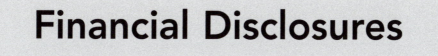

Financial Disclosures

Jeff Erickson, PT, MS, SCS, ATC, CSCS has no financial or proprietary interest in the materials presented herein.

Mia L. Erickson, PT, EdD, CHT, ATC has no financial or proprietary interest in the materials presented herein.

Rebecca McKnight, PT, MS has no financial or proprietary interest in the materials presented herein.

Tracy Rice, PT, MPH, NCS has no financial or proprietary interest in the materials presented herein.

Index